127 WILD MEDICINAL PLANTS OF SOUTHWESTERN US

GINA HOFFMAN

CONTENTS

INTRODUCTION

"Nature itself is the best physician." – Hippocrates.

You may be reading this book because you live, visit, hike, or forage in the Southwest. Or perhaps you (or a family member) have a medical problem and are looking into natural remedies and treatments. Many readers prefer to choose herbs and plants to improve their health rather than pay exorbitant prices for a packaged pill that may or may not help their symptoms and could cause side effects. Modern pharmaceutical drugs are costly, and their side effects can be severe. Some of you probably already use plants like herbs to make oils and preserve excess fruit in jams and cans for the winter months.

According to current research, even animals such as birds, elephants, and chimpanzees self-medicate[1]. For example, bears have been observed digging up skunk cabbage roots when they emerge from hibernation because the nutrient content is sufficient to help them when food is scarce and they are vulnerable. When animals are sick or weak, they eat specific plants to help them feel better, prevent disease, eliminate parasites, and aid digestion. Perhaps you've noticed this in your cat or dog.

Humans have looked to nature for powerful cures for their ailments since ancient times, creating remedies from wild plants and herbs growing nearby. Native Americans were the first to discover and use medicinal plants such as red clover, wild ginger, lavender, slippery elm, and many more. All of this knowledge and skill was passed down through family stories and traditional folklore to the next generation.

Despite the appearance that humans have lost touch with nature, this is not the case. Foraging for wild foods and using herbal plants are becoming more popular. Even if you are not a plant expert, you can still identify a stinging nettle and avoid it when walking through a forest. "If you are unfortunate enough to come across the stinging plant, you can employ an age-old herbal remedy with another commonly found forest plant. "The juice of a dock leaf can relieve nettle stings immediately."

Foraging in the wild or in your backyard and making a tincture is intriguing, but it may be more challenging than purchasing medication from a pharmacy. There are no labels, instructions, or pharmacists upon which to rely. What do I need? Where do I start? You have a lot of questions. I assume you've heard about some beneficial plants but aren't sure how to use them. You probably have some foraging skills and want to discover more ways to hone them. Foragers face the following difficulties:

- How do I recognize a plant? Is it toxic or medicinal?
- What, when, and how can I forage in my neighborhood?
- How should herbal medicines be made?
- What is the appropriate dose or measurement?

Before attempting to forage and use herbal remedies, it is critical to do some research to answer these questions. In this book, you will learn:

1. Over One Hundred Medicinal Plant Profiles: We will explore a variety of wild medicinal plants found in the American Southwest. These profiles give information about each plant, such as its scientific name, common name, range, preferred habitat, use, and side effects. You can also find QR codes containing scannable photo files.

2. The Rules of Foraging: You'll learn to practice responsible foraging with these ethical guidelines for harvesting wild herbs without harming the environment or breaking any laws. I've included a list of essential tools to have when foraging in the wild.

3. Plant Identification: Learn the fundamentals of identifying wild plants with pictures from six common plant families: aster, pea, mustard, parsley, and grass. We'll also cover the five key characteristics of poisonous plants and how to avoid them by following the eight golden rules of poison prevention.

4. How to Become a DIY Herbalist: Once you get your plant part safely home, there are guides on cleaning, drying, and preparing fantastic herbal recipes such as teas, tinctures, infusions, soothing balms, and baths.

GENERAL PRECAUTIONS

Before foraging medicinal herbs in the wild, be aware of the risks. While many plants benefit your health, others are poisonous and can have serious consequences. Because these toxic plants can look like herbs that are good for you, you must be careful about what you pick and eat. Even some medicinal plants can be harmful if not properly prepared and used. If you have a medical condition (including allergies) or are taking medication, it is always best to consult your doctor before using herbal remedies to avoid any interactions or unexpected side effects.

MY THOUGHTS AND EXPERIENCES

I believe nature can restore, sustain, and support us. For over fifteen years, I've been foraging locally, growing plants for my needs, and preparing herbal medicines. In my experience, when we take the time to slow down, notice the natural world around us, and respect the environment, we can recognize and appreciate more of nature's gifts.

Foraging for wild mushrooms and other plants was a big part of my childhood. As a child, my father would take us out in the woods and teach us how to identify and prepare them. In the spring, I would gather some young nettles to dry and make tea, infusions, and tinctures. I used to rinse my hair with nettle infusion. I count myself lucky to have learned the different uses of these plants at a young age.

Later in college, I studied biology, which inspired me to explore medicinal herbs more in depth. Over time, I accumulated a wealth of knowledge and began incorporating these practices into my daily life.

My goal with this book is to give you the confidence to go out into the wild as a forager and collect plants in your area. You, too, can learn to make home remedies and help your family live a healthier lifestyle while treating common ailments.

PART I

AN INTRODUCTION TO WILD MEDICINAL PLANTS

P lants have been used to aid in healing since the beginning of humankind. When herbs and local knowledge were the only medicines available, plants provide nourishment and kept people healthy. In the twenty-first century, it's difficult to imagine a world without hospitals, surgery, and anesthetics. But even modern drug companies agree that nature has given us a lot of things that are good for our bodies and can be used as medicines. They spend millions of dollars to find and test new parts of plants that can be used in supplements, drugs, and other treatments.

THE BENEFITS OF HERBAL MEDICINES

Medicinal plants have complex natural chemicals that the human body can't make or get from food, and each plant or herb has its own properties that can help your health in different ways. Skilled herbal practitioners diagnose patients based on physical exams, symptoms, lifestyle, and family history to find the root cause of illness, combine herbs, and make personalized medicine for each person.

Plants are the source of 11% of the 252 medications considered basic and essential for human health[1]. These include digoxin from the foxglove flower (*Digitalis* spp.), quinine, and quinidine from the cinchona tree bark (*Cinchona* spp.). Atropine comes from *Atropa belladonna,* and morphine and codeine come from the poppy (*Papaver somniferum*).

Herbal practitioners believe plant remedies are safe, effective, and have minimal adverse reactions. However, in some pharmaceutical drugs, only one active ingredient from natural plants is taken out and used in large doses. For example, the barks of meadowsweet (*Filipendula ulmaria*) and willow trees (*Salix sp.)* contain the salicylic acid used to make aspirin. Aspirin alone can cause the stomach lining to bleed, but the plant meadowsweet has other innate compounds that would stop salicylic acid from causing irritation. Thus, using the entire plant instead of just one part can be more beneficial.

One critical aspect of choosing plants for medicinal properties is that they grow locally; if you are confident in identifying them, these offer the most benefit for free.

Modern pharmaceutical drugs are also expensive, and herbal medicine is much more affordable. Another advantage of herbal medicine is that you do not need a doctor's prescription, so it is accessible to people who live in remote locations.

All over the world, natural herbal medicinal plants have been the first choice to treat illness. In some parts of the world, they still are. In Africa, reports from Ghana, Mali, and Zambia showed that more than half of the households asked were treating fever at home with herbal medicines.

HERBAL MEDICINES CONTAIN ACTIVE INGREDIENTS

Active ingredients are parts of herbs or plants that make the body react in a certain way. These substances also affect a plant's color, aroma, and flavor. They are also known as *phytochemicals*, and their job is to protect plants from drought, pollution, UV rays, and other environmental threats such as insect or pathogen attacks.

Phytochemicals are active substances found in plants that are beneficial when consumed by humans. Their primary function is to protect against damage or disease. Through scientific study, it has been found that phytochemicals are beneficial nutritionally and medicinally. Over 5000 phyto-chemicals have been found and cataloged[2]. These substances can be subdivided, and these headings are helpful if you want to understand how a particular plant can help you.

- **Adaptogenic**: *Adapt* means "to change something to suit a new circumstance." In terms of medicine, these herbs will help your body adapt to whatever health problem you have and can bring more balance to your body.
- **Anti-Inflammatory:** These are the plants that fight inflammation. When you hurt yourself, your body usually responds with swelling, pain, or redness in the area. Certain plants will reduce the swelling and relieve the pain. Some examples are black pepper (*Piper nigrum*), cardamom (*Elettaria*), garlic (Allium sativum), ginger (*Zingiber officinale*), ginseng (*Panax ginseng*), green tea(*Camellia sinensis*), rosemary (*Salvia rosemarius*), and turmeric (*Curcuma*).
- **Antimicrobial:** These plants actively fight bacteria or fungi. Examples are aloe (*Aloe vera*), cloves (*Syzygium aromaticum*), garlic, sage (*Salvia officinalis*), and thyme (*Thymus vulgaris*).
- **Antioxidant:** Plants that stop or reduce the effect of free radicals in the body fall into this category. Examples include turmeric, yarrow(*Achillea millefolium*), garlic, coriander (*Coriandrum sativum*), ginger, and ginseng.

- **Antiviral:** This means that a plant increases or boosts immunity against specific viruses or conditions like the common cold, influenza, etc. Some examples are tulsi (*Ocimum tenuiflorum*) leaves, black pepper, ginger , cinnamon (*Cinnamomum verum*), and guduchi (*Tinospora cordifolia*).
- **Nootropic plants:** These plants effectively enhance memory and support cognitive health. Some examples are bacopa (*Bacopa monnieri*), ginkgo (*Ginkgo biloba*), gotu kola (*Centella asiatica*), lemon balm (*Melissa officinalis*), and rosemary.

HERBAL PREPARATION BASICS

The herbal practitioner may prescribe the following methods of preparation and administration of medicinal plants:

- Herbal infusions use fresh or dried leaves, flowers, fruits, bark, stems, or roots.
- Fresh leaves are eaten as food in salads or cooked and added to dishes.
- Fresh leaves are used as a poultice directly on the skin.
- Fresh or dried flowers are eaten or used in oils and infusions.
- Fruit (e.g., rosehips) can be dried and grated for teas and made into syrup and jelly.

- Tinctures are made using plants seeped in oil to extract the goodness, and drops of this concentrated herb are diluted with water.
- Use salve or ointment to heal an infected wound, sting, or burn.
- Grated roots are eaten or used in food (e.g., ginger or dandelion root).

MEDICINAL BENEFIT OF SPECIFIC PLANTS

Herbal medicine has used the plants below for hundreds of years, and there has been much research and testing on how they improve health. The following are some examples of beneficial plants used in herbal and conventional medicine:

Gallega officinalis

Over 400 plant-derived products have been used worldwide to treat late-onset diabetes (Type 2). Goat's rue (*Gallega officinalis*) has the active ingredient galegine, which is used in the most effective treatments. Galegine was used to create metformin, which is used to treat late-onset diabetes worldwide. This medicine greatly lowers blood sugar levels, and when combined with a healthy lifestyle, it improves health in general.

Echinacea angustifolia

Echinacea (*Echinacea angustifolia*) is used to aid the body's immune system. It can be used topically on boils and stimulates the immune system.

Allium sativum

Garlic (*Allium sativum*) Garlic is proven to lower cholesterol in the blood and support heart function. It has been shown to reduce the growth of bacteria when used in packaging, and it is antiviral, working against colds and flu.

Zingiber officinale

Ginger root (*Zingiber officinale*) has been used to treat all kinds of nausea, from morning sickness to motion sickness to nausea caused by viruses and inflammation.

Hypericum perforatum

St. John's Wort (*Hypericum perforatum*) can help relieve anxiety and sleeplessness, and it can also be used to treat mild depression. Be careful. It interferes with other drugs (e.g., the contraceptive pill), so consult your medical professional.

Cinchona officinalis

Quinine (*Cinchona officinalis*) is used to treat fever and malaria. It was "found" in Peru, where it was historically used for this function by the Quechua Indians. The World Health Organization's most recommended and effective malaria treatment, quinine, is made from an infusion of the bark of the Cinchona tree. This medication is available locally, is less expensive, and is more sustainable for those who have practical knowledge of plants for medicine.

Artemisia annua

Sweet Annie (*Artemisia annua*) is a Chinese sagebrush used for centuries to cure malaria and infectious diarrhea. The World Health Organization (WHO) has recognized a chemical called *artemisinin*, present in the leaves of this plant, as helpful in treating malaria[3]. It is usually preserved in a tincture and taken with water.

Prosopis glandulosa

If you live in the southwestern United States, you're probably familiar with the beautiful Texas native mesquite tree (*Prosopis glandulosa*) (see page 188). Native Americans have eaten this plant for centuries. The sweet-flavored pods are ground into flour using stone tools. When protein is scarce, the seeds' high protein content supplements diets. The medicinal value of both the bark and the leaves is less known. Historically, the inner bark was removed and processed to be used as a laxative (or an emetic). The leaves were combined with water to make a tea to treat stomach pain and an eyewash for sore eyes.

Typha

Cattail (*Typha*) (see page 133) is another common plant in the United States, with a southern variety growing in Arizona. Cattails can remove heavy metals and toxins from the water that tend to lodge in the plant and are indicators of environmental pollution.

Native Americans ate pollen, flowers, young shoots, and roots throughout the year. These roots produced a large amount of flour, which was stored for the winter and could be used as an emergency bandage in remote areas to stop bleeding. A small section of the root was dug out and cut in half, then applied directly to the wound as an antiseptic.

SPECIAL CONSIDERATIONS

Taking herbal medicine (or supplements) may increase or decrease the effectiveness of other drugs or increase the risk of adverse side effects from using them with chemical pharmaceuticals. If you are thinking about using herbal remedies, discuss with your doctor and a herbalist about any potential side effects.

Furthermore, you should never pick your plants without first considering the area's safety. For example, I would never tell you to gather plants from the side of a road in a city where herbicides or weed killers may have been used.

HOW OFTEN SHOULD HERBAL MEDICINE BE TAKEN?

If you have an herbal prescription, follow the dosage recommendations and take it as directed by your herbal practitioner. For example, they may tell you only to take three cups of tea daily because the side effects of the tea may outweigh the benefits if taken more than the prescribed number of times. Or the prescription might be a teaspoonful of a particular oil or a certain number of drops of a tincture added to a glass of water.

Eating fresh herbs or using ginger as a seasoning will add health benefits to your meals. Remember that herbal medicines may take longer than prescribed antibiotics or prescriptions. Be patient and allow time for the plant to do its work. Compare it with how plants grow in the wild. It takes time for the plant to absorb water via its roots or sunlight via its leaves. The same principle applies to you.

You undoubtedly understand that medicinal herbs are more beneficial than conventional medicine. In the following chapters, you will learn that there are many ways to use wild medicinal plants and many ways to make natural medicines from them. Before you run out with a bag to pick every wild plant you know, read the foraging principles for sustainable foraging.

GUIDELINES FOR ETHICAL AND SUSTAINABLE FORAGING

W hen you understand how beneficial plant medicine is, you might feel compelled to go out and collect some plants the next day. However, Mother Nature would have very little left if the entire world started to forage tomorrow. This chapter will teach you how to harvest plants safely and sustainably so that you can continue to enjoy them for years to come.

WHAT IS ETHICAL FORAGING?

Foraging is gathering wild fruits, leaves, fungi, roots, bark, and other things to eat or make into food or medicine. Ethical foraging means collecting mindfully and foraging with gratitude and respect. In ethical foraging, it is important to pay attention to the environment, not just for what one can collect but also for the ecological balance of the ecosystem. Foraging in this manner ensures long-term sustainability.

Imagine yourself as a gatherer of plants when there was no refrigeration, but you needed to use them out of season. You'd probably know the area well, have chosen the correct harvest season, and have decided where to find your desired plants in abundance. You would see the plant you are looking for and cut several leaves, dig out a little of the root, or take a small amount of the bark.

It's crucial to keep in mind that wild medicinal plants are an important part of our natural environment and that they should be treated with care and respect. A responsible forager will notice any damage to the plant. When digging a hole for root collection, the ethical thing to do is to ensure the remaining plant has enough roots to survive and then fill the void with soil.

Native Americans have harvested wild plants for thousands of years while still honoring the landscape. They ensure that cuts made to tree bark only happen for a certain period and that enough berries are left for birds and wildlife. Respect for the natural environment and gratitude for the harvest are inherent to their collecting practices.

RULES TO CONSIDER

1. Plan Your Foraging Trip

Before you set off, you must have a plan. Make a list of everything you need. You'll need a good guidebook, the right tools, an emergency first aid kit, and a collecting bag to keep your foraged material safe until you get home. Fully charge your mobile and inform someone exactly where you intend to look for plants. Adding a phone number for the local hospital, your health care provider, or somebody to call in an emergency is a good idea.

Drinking water is essential, particularly in hot weather. You are often alone in the wild, and the weather can change dramatically. Always check the weather forecast. Bring your medication if you have an allergy or medical condition. You can then relax, knowing that you have done everything you need to do before going outside to connect with nature.

2. Only Pick What You Need

If you see several different plants growing, pick a few parts from each and store them well in your collection bag. The general rule is to harvest between one-tenth and one-third for yourself, leaving one-third for the environment and one-third for the plant. This allows birds and wildlife to live on it, the plant to grow, and some herbs in your bag.

Remember that if you harvest all the flowers in the spring from one plant, the cut flowers cannot make fruit that forms in the fall. You risk killing a plant if you remove all of its leaves. Do not pick it if it is the sole plant in the area.

Do not pick from a single plant if it is the only one of its type. Try to find a patch of plants growing together, and then do not choose unhealthy or diseased leaves. If you plan on removing some bark or cutting a branch, only take what you need and replace the outer bark.

3. Check for identification.

Before harvesting a plant, you must double-check at least three points of identification. These can include flower, leaf size, shape, stem, color, season, smell, and bark. Remember that plants look different in each season.

Invest in good guidebooks, and when you see new, unfamiliar plants, try to identify them from the book. Take photographs of unknown plants and post them on online community forums. It allows other people to help you identify the plant.

Another great idea is to join a community group to learn from experts. There are guided walks with experts who can give you confidence and show you any well-known poisonous plants. They can usually explain where to find the plants and how to choose them, as they know the local paths and the flowering or fruiting times.

4. Get the Right Tools and Equipment

Foraging is typically done on foot, so consider this when purchasing tools. They must be of high quality, lightweight, and user-friendly. Wooden-handled trowels are my favorite, and I've had the same one for 15 years, so investing in quality tools is worthwhile. Sharpen your pruners or knives to make clean cuts and avoid any damage. Please scan the QR code below to find some photos of hand tool requirements.

- **Clothing:** Your clothes must be suitable for striding through nettles, brambles, and poison ivy (maybe even a swarm of bees). Wear long-sleeved tops, long pants, closed-toe shoes or boots, thick socks, and a good hat for shade and protection (with a veil) in overgrown areas where some plants may be poisonous.
- **Gardening Gloves:** It's best to wear long-sleeved leather gloves and disposable or washable rubber gloves when working with plants you don't know much about. When completed, change your gloves and place them in a plastic bag in your collecting bag. Make sure you clean these afterward at home.

- **Magnifying Glass or Camera:** Sometimes, it isn't easy to measure or inspect a plant part with the naked eye, and a magnifying glass can help with this. An alternative method is to snap a photo on your phone and enlarge it so you can view it in more detail. Put a portion of your hand in the image to judge size accurately.

- **Measuring Device:** Use a ruler with both inches and metric measurements. You will also need a measuring tape to measure trees. This is super useful because you can place a leaf there to check the leaf's expected size or the stem's width.

- **Record-Keeping Supplies:** Recording the date and the area is helpful for every expedition. A photo of every plant collected will accurately record the date and time. Sometimes you will want to write extra notes to aid conservation records. Sticky labels can be added to containers (see more below) if you have any doubts about identification.

- **Pocket Knife:** A knife is often helpful when cutting a thick stem or leaf. Ensure it is sharpened before you go, or you will damage the plants. Some knives have fixed blades with a sheath cover to protect you when you are not using them. The traditional Japanese garden knife, Hori-Hori, is also handy, especially for digging and cutting roots.

- **Pruning Saw:** Most of these are small and easy to carry. Some come with a blade cover, which is great if it fits in your foraging pack. When slicing thorny twigs or stems, use these. To minimize accidental damage when foraging, get a saw with a safety catch or lock.

- **Pruning Shears:** The best ones have extendable arms that can reach up to high branches out of your reach, which is helpful for fruit collection or pruning back an overgrown shrub. Be mindful not to cut at random; use these to cut edible flowers, shoots, leaves, and stems, and make the first cut to collect bark. Higher grades are made of rust-resistant stainless steel, and many come with a safety catch that locks the blades when not in use.

- **Scissors:** Buy a heavyweight pair of scissors that you can use to cut leaves, stems, and flowers at ground level. These need to be heavyweight, and I do not recommend using a set from your first aid kit for fear of poison contamination from plant to wound. Have some wipes or antiseptic cleaner to wipe them down if you pick up anything that may be poisonous.

- **Trowel and Hand Shovel:** When you're foraging, having a good-quality trowel with a wooden handle is helpful. This is because you often have to check roots underground or dig up a part of the root. Dig carefully to avoid ruining the root system, and clean down the trowel with a cloth if you are digging for anything that may be poisonous. It is not practical to carry a full-sized shovel, but you will find sets of trowels and hand shovels in most gardening or camping stores. Try to choose something lightweight but comfortable.

- **Airtight Containers or Collecting Bags:** Conserving anything you pick is essential. Collecting bags made of natural, breathable materials are often the best. If it is a warm summer day, you may want to add some cool packs from your freezer to conserve leaves. Keep plants in separate containers with sticky labels. You should recycle some food containers with lids for foraging. These can be scrubbed, dried, and reused time after time. Glass jars with lids are also helpful and environmentally friendly. However, these can break, and recycled plastic is lighter.
- **First-Aid Kit:** It would be best if you had some plasters, bandages, alcohol wipes, hand sanitizer, painkillers, and small scissors, as well as an antibacterial ointment for wounds. Other things like a flashlight, a lighter, safety pins, sticky tape, and a whistle are also important. Keep in mind your foraging trip time and the location's season., and always remember the emergency contact numbers.

5. Legal and Ethical Foraging Requires Permission and Respect

This is the first thing you should address on your foraging list. Is it lawful to choose the region where you wish to collect? Overcollection in the United States has damaged certain herbal plants. Individuals buy them at health food shops and then harvest their own in the wild. A good source for learning about endangered plant species is the United Plant Savers website, which includes a 3-category list of wild medicinal plants identified as threatened or endangered in North America[1]. If the plant is on the list, buy and plant seeds at home. American ginseng, white sage, cascara sagrada, echinacea, osha, slippery elm, spikenard, yerba mansa, and more plants are all on the "at-risk" list.

It is also important to remember that you cannot just decide to forage on private property. If you do, you may be fined. It is always much better to talk to the landowner, who may let you on their land in exchange for some of your plants or volunteer work on wildlife tasks. You must check local parks' legalities with your municipality's parks and recreation office. The Forest Service can tell you if foraging is permitted in parks and how much is allowed. Find a local fisherman or ask at an angler's shop if you want to take plants from the water. Where fishermen go, the water is safe for fish, which is usually an excellent place to pick plants. You will also need to see if any possible pollutants are present.

6. Only Harvest From a Safe, Unpolluted Area

Observe bugs and wildlife as you explore an area. You may surprise a sunbathing lizard or find caterpillars munching on leaves. Evidence of nature is good news because it shows the whole area is a living habitat. Observe how the site is managed on your regular walks. Roadside plants may be sprayed as part of the management plan. Weeds must be controlled, especially in industrial areas, along the edges of busy roads, and even in city park shrubs. If you meet one of these people spraying, note down the name of the weed killer and research its chemicals.

If you are unsure about a property line or any chemical sprays that may have been used, avoid the area. Plants take in chemicals, pollutants, heavy metals, and other harmful things through their roots. This is known as bioaccumulation. Walk a bit before picking. If you meet another forager, ask them for advice. They may know the area better than you and can teach you which plants are in season and which should be avoided. Keep your eyes peeled for any significant changes. If a large area, typically green, has brown or blackened leaves, this is a good indicator that somebody has sprayed a chemical to kill them, and it is not a good place to forage. There may be a simple explanation, such as severe drought or the end of the plant's cycle, but it is best to be safe.

If you forage in an urban area, finding foraging sites can be as easy as searching the internet! Falling fruit is a database of over half a million food sources worldwide in urban areas.

7. Leave the Area in the Same (or Better) Condition Than You Found It

See yourself as a guardian of all the spaces you walk in. If you believe that every plant, creature, and element of this landscape affects your foraged plants' health, you will stay attuned to any changes. Protect all aspects of nature within your foraging area. For example, ants clean up the soil and bring seeds into the ground; worms fertilize and make air vents in the earth; caterpillars grow into the gorgeous butterflies that pollinate our flowers; and ladybugs eat harmful insects.

If you have young foragers with you, teach them never to kill a bug or a caterpillar and explain how it is part of a food cycle. Even slugs and snails recycle fallen leaves and clean the soil surface into usable, rich soil for the following year's plant growth. If there is water, don't throw anything dirty in it, potentially interfering with the wildlife.

As you walk, pick up bottles or trash that people have thrown away. Have a collection bag for foraged material and a separate bag for trash. Try not to drive off-road. Your feet will not cause significant damage, but the wheels of a 4x4 can crush both plants and wildlife and change a whole area. If you bring food or drinks, take the trash home with you. Try to leave your walk the same as you found it. If there is a way to improve it, then by all means, do so. Please do not change the environment drastically; try to leave it cleaner and happier for your visit.

8. Observe and Give Back

You become closer to the natural world when you venture out for a foraging walk. You start to feel the wind in your hair and the sun on your skin. As the paths you regularly walk become more familiar, you will notice signs of the changing seasons. The blooms change, new buds open, and the temperature changes. A forager must become familiar with and aware of their local area. You may find yourself concerned because one of your favorite plants did not bloom. There could be an innocent reason, such as bad weather. Or perhaps you notice a potential issue, such as an invasive weed like Japanese knotweed taking over an area. Issues such as this can be dealt with when responsible foragers notify local authorities.

What does it mean to give back? As mentioned earlier, it might mean noticing an invasive plant and telling an authority. It might mean picking up the mess that someone else has left. It could be collecting seeds and taking a few home (if permitted in your state) or scattering them at a distance from the mother plant so that they can grow in another spot. If you dig a hole, fill it back in before you leave. If you have extra water and a plant looks very dry, spill a small amount from your bottle. This is particularly important after digging a root because it will help the root settle in. Foragers can help promote balance by spreading seeds or runners of endangered plants and harvesting from more plentiful plants. Online conservation campaigns reach and educate many more people than word-of-mouth, so if you are good at technology, this can be your contribution. Look into volunteering or fundraising for your local park or wildlife area.

A further way to give back to nature is to learn together, share your experiences in a group, and spread ethical foraging practices in the community.

IN CONCLUSION

Know your area—your back and front gardens. Become familiar with your regular walking routes. You will be amazed at how much you can learn in just one year by listening to experts, a local forager, or somebody who loves wildflowers or butterflies. Eventually, you will start to notice new shoots and surprise yourself by knowing what they are and if they are safe to pick. No matter what you observe, the point is that you are becoming more aware of the natural world. Record your experience in some way so that it can be shared.

This is part of our path as natural world keepers, or stewards. Respect it, enjoy it, and pass it on to someone else. Sharing what you know helps to improve the environment around you. You can volunteer to count birds, beetles, or butterflies on national counting survey days, or you can become a plant observer who tells the authorities when a new plant grows. Perhaps your home garden or balcony will be brimming with seeds and plants, never disappointing you.

Practice the principles of ethical foraging. Never pick too much; the plant must survive if you want to keep harvesting for many more years. Once you understand how to safely and responsibly forage wild plants, you can be more confident when it comes to using them.

Going forward, you need to know how to avoid any plants that may be poisonous. We will cover this in the next chapter, where you will learn how to stay safe while in the wild.

SAFETY CONSIDERATIONS WHEN FORAGING

This chapter will review some safety precautions to ensure your foraging trips don't end in disaster. Before foraging, it is essential to research the area and be aware of any potentially dangerous plants, fungi, or animals.

HOW TO IDENTIFY POISONOUS PLANTS

Foraging plants and mushrooms for food and medicine in the wild has become popular in recent years. According to the American Association of Poison Control Centers (AAPCC), this practice causes an increase in foraging accidents and fatalities. Plants can be poisonous either by touch or by ingestion. When foraging for plants and mushrooms, keep the following three things in mind:

1. Accidentally eating poisonous plants and plant parts happens when collecting and consuming unidentified poisonous plants and mushrooms.
2. Don't eat and use plants contaminated by harmful chemicals like pesticides, herbicides, and other toxins. Forage in unpolluted safe areas; stay away from roadside and industrial areas.
3. Allergic reactions to some plants, even edible ones, happen. Every plant has many active chemical compounds, and the human body can respond differently. It can cause an allergic reaction. If you try new plants, eat small amounts first and wait 24 hours to see if there is any reaction.

Several indicators are common for toxic plants. Here are five warning signs to keep an eye out for:

- white or milky-white colored sap (from a cut stem, leaf, or any part of the plant)
- yellow and white berries, and sometimes green
- umbel-shaped plants
- glossy green or dull leaves
- a single leaf, with three leaflets – 3 leaf pattern growth

Milky sap is usually found in the stem or when you cut a leaf or a branch, but remember to wear gloves to protect yourself before cutting anything. The first forager's rule is that milky sap is often poisonous, so if you notice it, move on.

Yellow and white berries appear on many poisonous plants. Generally, you should assume that these berries are all poisonous. Botanists agree that at least 85–90% of all white or yellow berries are dangerous for humans, although some animals or birds may be able to consume them. Doll's eyes, white sumac, and poison oak are poisonous and possibly fatal. Some red berries, such as those of holly, ivy, mistletoe, and yew, are also toxic. Red, blue, and blackberries are more likely to be palatable if they do not grow in bunches—for example, blackberries and strawberries. Pokeberry is the exception; it is toxic and should never be eaten. A bunch of berries is less likely to be edible, so think of elderberries growing in a cluster with a deep black color, which is not safe raw but is fine when cooked. Remember that there may be exceptions to every rule, so the best way to identify poisonous plants is to learn them from an expert guide and use this book.

Use caution with **flowering umbels.** Umbel refers to the shape of the flowering head; think of an upside-down umbrella with a similar profile. The stalks are linked together by a central point. The stalks are usually the same length, and the "umbrella" shape can be flat or curved, just like an umbrella. Elderflowers are edible, but elderberries that form later need to be cooked before you eat them. Carrot umbels are the seeds of the vegetable, but poison hemlock also has umbels. If you are in any doubt, leave them be.

Look for **glossy green or dull leaves**. The edges of the leaf tend to have a pointed edge pattern, and the leaves themselves are smooth. Poison oak is a good example; the common stinging nettle is another.

Beware **a single leaf with three leaflets**—the three-leaf pattern of growth. "Leaves of three, let it be," as the proverb goes, and if one leaf stands straight while the others are on the left and right, you should not choose this plant. Poison ivy and poison oak have the same appearance[1]. These indications suggest you should never include this leaf in your foraging bag. Poison sumac is an exception, as it has multiple leaves (up to 13) bunched together and is not in the 3-leaf pattern; therefore, be cautious. Each plant you pick may be an exception, and you must have a positive ID before harvesting it.

Remember, some plants have poisonous look-alikes! Some plants, at a glance, look similar to others. For example, giant hogweed and cow parsnip are in the same parsley family, but giant hogweed is poisonous while cow parsnip is edible. The flower shape is similar; the important identification keys are the leaf shape, size, stem color, and hair. Poisonous pokeweed (*Phytolacca americana*) berries are similar in color and shape to elderberries (*Sambucus*) and grow in the same habitat. The difference is that berries are unlikely to appear on the leaves.

Please scan the QR code below to view photos of poisonous plants!

Additional clues that may indicate poison include:

- spines and small, pointy hairs on the leaf's surface (Think of a stinging nettle!)
- bitter or soapy taste and smell (These smells are a warning!)
- spurs, spikes, or thorns (These are often a sign that you should keep away, especially if they are pink, black, or purple.)

HOW DO POISONOUS PLANTS AFFECT US?

Poisonous plants affect our bodies in four different ways. Some are merely inconvenient, but some are fatal if not treated urgently! Symptoms may not show until hours later.

Plants Affecting the Skin

Remember that some plant parts may be edible, but others may contain poison. All parts of the dandelion are edible except the sap, which can be used externally on warts but shouldn't be consumed. For example, see comfrey, stinging nettles, poison hemlock, oleander, manchineel, monkshood, prickly pear cactus, poison ivy, poison sumac, poison oak, and wild parsnip.

Plants Affecting the Digestive System

Some plants have toxic properties that affect the digestive system. Symptoms include nausea, vomiting, abdominal pain, diarrhea, and primary organ failure. For example, see castor beans, poison oak, elderberry, manchineel, water hemlock, iris, pokeweed, rosary pea, white snakeroot, and deadly nightshade.

Plants Affecting the Nervous System

Severe symptoms after consumption of these plants can include total collapse, seizures, and paralysis. The person may become unresponsive to touch or sound. One example would be an angel's trumpet.

Plants Affecting the Heart

Plants may cause a faster or slower heartbeat than usual, you may have difficulty breathing, and you may have cramps or other symptoms. These plants may not affect you immediately. Some symptoms may take 24 hours to occur. Report difficulty breathing or drops in blood pressure to a medical professional. Monkshood, foxglove, and oleander are examples of this plant category.

EMERGENCY FIRST AID: IF YOU COME INTO CONTACT WITH A POISONOUS PLANT

Before you set out, ensure you have a first aid kit with outdoor skin protection or Tecnu for cleansing. Include a phone number for local poison control and a doctor's or hospital's phone number for any area where you will be staying. In an emergency, this extra effort could save your life. Several pairs of polythene gloves are helpful if you need to treat poison. It is because simply touching some poisons is dangerous, and you do not want to transfer the poison to anyone not affected. Have a separate bag for waste, such as used cotton balls and gloves.

- If you come into contact with poison ivy, poison oak, or any other poisonous plants that affect the skin and develop a rash, immediately rinse your skin with rubbing alcohol, Tecnu wash, soapy water, or even clear water.
- Rince it often. Make sure you do not use this same cotton ball again. Have a trash bag, insert used items, and avoid touching anything with poison.
- Scrub under nails with a brush.
- Apply hydrocortisone cream, and take antihistamines, if available, to reduce irritation.
- Cold compresses also help; just be careful not to apply them too long and avoid direct contact with the skin. Oatmeal baths relieve itches and redness.

- If you can do this safely, use tweezers to remove prickly thorns, and save these in a bag or tissue to show a medical professional later.
- Call the doctor if the rash spreads and develops into a fever or if you have breathing difficulties, hives, and swelling.

If anything you have eaten makes you feel sick or nauseous, make yourself vomit, rinse your mouth with water, and then spit this out. Do this twice. Then drink some water to rehydrate your body.

Immediately call emergency services and seek professional help if you have severe symptoms like difficulty breathing, heart rate changes, vomiting, diarrhea, or a seizure with paralysis.

THE EIGHT GOLDEN RULES OF POISON PREVENTION

The rules are simple, but you must follow them to stay safe. Native Americans prepare very carefully for a trip into the wild, and some have amulets with them as a reminder that each leaf or berry picked comes from a live plant, thanks must be given, and they must take no more than is needed.

The 8 Golden Rules

1. **Know your plants.** Research before you go and know what you are looking for. Make a positive ID from a book, chart, or phone before picking.

2. **Don't eat unknown plants, mushrooms, or berries.** If you cannot positively identify the plant, leaf, or berry, check for similar-looking ones in your book, and do not eat anything until you are 100% sure it matches all descriptions. Check the leaf size, stem thickness, flowers (if applicable), and any notes about the plant. I usually place everything in my collecting bag and wait until I get home to be sure. Some plants and fruits must be cooked before they are safe, so check which part is edible and follow the instructions.

3. **Dress properly.** It would be best to have long trousers or pants, a long-sleeved top, and gloves. Thick fabrics are recommended.

4. **Wash your hands and clothing after touching them.** If you have handled unknown plants on your walk, carefully clean your hands and skin with soap and water on arrival home and wash your clothes before you wear them again.

5. **Protect your pets.** Some plant leaves are not harmful to humans but may adversely affect pets. When you come home, wash your hands before you stroke or pet an animal.

6. **Be cautious when burning unknown plants.** Many plants like lavender, bay, or rosemary burn beautifully as kindling for bonfires. Check the smoke is not hazardous before using any unknown wood. Avoid inhaling smoke. Manchineel is a good example. If it gets in your eyes, you could lose your eyesight. Eating the fruit is fatal. See more in Appendix, Table 1 (page 51)

7. **Avoid making items.** It will seem harsh to those who love making daisy chains, but if you have chosen a poisonous plant or fruit, the poison may transfer to your hands or skin. This means not making necklaces or bracelets until you have identified every plant you want to use.

8. **Carry decontaminating wash, e.g., Tecnu, and a proper first aid kit.** If you discover that you have touched something dangerous, always have a supply of decontaminating wash to clean the affected area as soon as possible. One example of a plant that is not always harmful (depending on the individual) are comfrey leaves. They are harmless to most but can cause a rash in others. Keep supplies on hand to rinse any unexpected irritations.

TIPS FOR SUCCESS

- **Talk to a local expert** to identify the plant if you can. Try to forage with someone who knows the area and its plants. If you are alone in the field, you could snap a photo and send it to somebody to assess if you are in a group. Then, talk to the person with the most expertise and listen to what they say. Local experts will know all the tricks to safely identify, pick, eat, and prepare. Click on the link below to find experienced foragers in your area if you want to join a local foraging group. https://www.robgreenfield. org/findaforager

- **Some so-called "experts" may not be.** It may go against the previous rule, but don't drink it until you're confident it's been identified. Create a checklist. Recognize the distinguishing characteristics. Share a picture in groups online; if it is poisonous, someone will usually respond. However, in a life-or-death situation, you can only depend on yourself.

- **Know your chosen place.** Private property should be respected, and foraging should be legal. Some states have strict rules about what you can collect and when you can collect it. If you find edible or medicinal plants in polluted areas, do not pick them. Pesticides or herbicides may be present if the land has been treated. When it rains, chemicals run into neighboring streams and pollute them. Never go scavenging near a dump!

- **Use your senses in this order: see, smell, hear, touch, and taste.** Look at the plant to identify it correctly. Color can also determine the likelihood of poisoning. A bitter smell can often indicate that the plant is unsafe for you. The stinking lily is so named for its horrible odor, which warns you that the bulb is poisonous. Sound is interesting because gorse makes a crackling sound in the fall; this is a seed dispersal method. Some trees make a specific sound when the wind blows through their leaves; you can be sure it is that tree because of the sound. This is known as *psithurism*. For example, pine trees sound different from the sound of the wind rustling the leaves of an oak or willow. Could you go out and listen to it? Do not touch unless you are entirely sure. In an emergency, cover your hand with clothing or a cloth bag before touching a plant. Assess if the plant has milky sap or if the stem or leaf is hairy. Your skin will react if you touch a stinging plant, like a nettle. Only taste after you have tried looking, smelling, listening, and touching. Then do a skin and lip test before you swallow that leaf or berry.

- **Use it only if you can check off every item on your checklist.** Remember the five characteristic signs of poisonous plants!
- **Mushrooms are not safe.** Of course, there are some safe mushrooms. Mushrooms are not plants; they are fungi. Do not eat any mushrooms if you are the slightest bit unsure. Some are toxic, and eating one

alone in the wild could be fatal. Some are also known to be hallucinogenic and medicinal.

- **Animals eat plants, so I can eat them too!** This is not the case. Some birds can eat holly and ivy berries, but humans cannot. Humans have different digestive systems than animals. Just because you see an animal ingest a plant does not mean it is safe for you.

- **Also, keep in mind that plants that smell like onions are safe.** The smell is a positive identifier. If it looks like an onion and smells like an onion, it is an onion. Chives, onions, leeks, and garlic all have this unmistakable smell. Break off a bit of the leaf stem, which should identify it safely. A lily that grows in Florida looks like an onion, but it does not have the smell, so your nose would correctly identify that it is not an onion. That lily is called crow poison or false onion,(*Nothoscordum bivalve*) which is a toxic look-alike of wild onion, but you would not try to eat it because it does not smell like an onion.

- **All plants in the mustard family (*Brassicaceae*) are edible.** It is safe if you are confident that you can identify the plant as part of this family. (See page 58.) Growing it at home is the best way to familiarize yourself with this plant. Growing a plant gives you a lot more awareness, so when you are out in the wild, you will recognize the seed or head of the flower (depending on the season), and you can use this experience to identify it. Mustard seeds are available to buy in seed stores and can be grown at home, too, so you get used to the leaf's shape, the flowers' color, and the height it grows.

- **The smell test works on mints too.** Use your sense of smell; mint smells the same in almost every country. Tear a leaf from the stem, and the smell should be unmistakable. There are 600 varieties of mint worldwide. There is spearmint, peppermint, apple mint, and so on. All of them are edible if they smell like mint. However, be careful. Some people have a strong allergy to mint, so if you are one of them, do not eat this plant.

This chapter has taught you about the dangers that may be hiding in plants that grow nearby. The main takeaways are: Forage safely! Do not touch any plants unless you are 100% sure. Also, you should seek expert advice and join a foraging group when you first start. Wear appropriate clothing and use GPS maps, the right tools, and your first-aid kit.

Once you understand how to safely and responsibly forage wild plants, you can be more confident when it comes to using them.

APPENDIX

Table 1. Common poisonous plants of the Southwestern region

	Names of poisonous plants	Poisonous part(s)	Body part it affects	Symptoms	Distribution or habitat
1	Castor beans-Ricinus communis	Seed, Sap contains a toxin called -risin	Digestive system, skin rash, also can get allergic reaction	Fatal; nausea, diarrhea, heart palpitation, low blood pressure seizures	Cultivated but grows in the wild
2	Corn cockle-Agrostem ma githago	all parts of the plant	digestive system, liver damage	gastric pain, diarrhea	Throughout most of the country fields, roadside and disturbed areas
3	Cow parsnip-Heracleu m maximum	sap	skin nervous system	cause photosensitivi ty and dermatitis	the country. grows woodlands,gras sland waterside and roadside
4	Chinaberry-Melia azedarach	fruits	nervous system	loss appetite, stomach discomfort,dia rrhea disorientation, weakness	widely spread in southern states, roadside
5	Deadly Nightshade Belladonna-Atrop a belladonna	All parts	digestive system, heart, nervous system,even complication of pregnancy	headache,blur red vision,heart palpitations,lo ss of balance,consti pation ,hallucination	shady moist areas, disturbed soils
6	Death Camas(meadow) -Toxicoscordion venenosum	All parts	digestive system, mussels,respirato ry system, nervous system	vomiting,mus cle weakness, tremors,convu lsion, coma and death	Native in western North America, dry meadow, sandy hillsides and mountain forest
7	Elderberry-Samb ucus	Raw berries and another part of the plant contain toxins	digestive system,	Nausea, vomiting, cramps, diarrhea	widespread throughout US, grows anywhere sunny places
8	Water hemlock -Cicuta	All parts, roots are most toxic in early spring	nervous system	nausea, vomiting, tremors seizures, death	widespread in the US, growing in alongside water or swamps and in water

9	Jimson weed-Datura stramonium	All parts of the plant	Nervous system	delirium,hallu cination,bizarr e behavior,amn esia	Native to North America
10	Jack-in-pulpit-Arisaema triphyllum	All parts	mouth, digestive system	Mouth, and throat irritation,	Native in Eastern North America. (Texas) moist woodlands
11	Larkspur -Delphinium nuttallii, and bicolour	All parts of the plant	Heart and nervous, and digestive systems	severe digestive discomfort, skin irritation	all through US mountain meadow, prairie
12	Manchineel-Hipp omane mancinella	Sap, leaves, the fruit, and smoke from burning wood Mexico, it	Skin. Eyes. Digestive tract. Smoke – affects the eyes and lungs	Blisters. It can cause blindness. Lung problems.	tropical of the South US. Mostly sandy beaches
13	Monkshood-Acon itum	Whole plant. The sap in the eyes causes blindness.	Skin, Heart. Eyes.	Nausea, vomiting, diarrhea, sweating, dizziness, and difficulty breathing death	throughout mountainous parts of the country. (mountain meadows)
14	Moonflower-Ipomoea alba	All parts	nervous system, digestive system, and bladder	hallucinogenic effect, nausea, thirst, and dry mouth,	Southwest as a weed in ditches and roadsides
15	Texas Mountain Laurel Dermatophyllum secundiflorum	(all parts of plants are toxic)	if consuming single seed	Difficulty breathing,nau sea vomiting, dizziness, heart failure, death	Native to Texas and New Mexico, it grows in rocky soils.
16	Poison Oak-Toxicodendron diversilobum	Leaves and twigs contain oil urushiol which causes contact dermatitis	Allergic reaction to the skin, the smoke can poison	Redness, rash on the skin, itchiness, blisters	South California,, grassland, oak woodland, and mixed evergreen forest
17	Poison ivy-Toxicodendro n radicans, rydbergii	Leaves. Contact with plants on the skin. (urushiol)	Allergic reaction to the skin, the smoke can poison	Redness, rash on skin Irritation, blisters	throughout the US. Grows along waterside(river , lake, beaches)
18	Wild Poinsettia-Eupho rbia heterophylla	All part	Skin, some people get allergic reaction	Skin rashes, swelling, nausea, shortness of breath...	subtropic and tropic, desert area

4

IDENTIFYING MEDICINAL PLANTS IN THE WILD

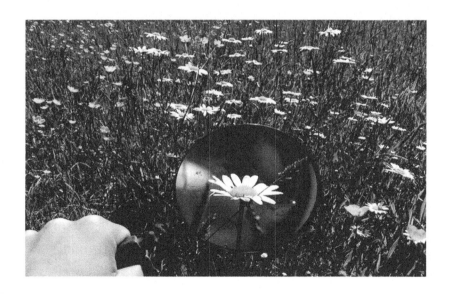

P lant identification is an essential foraging, gardening, and survival skill. Remember that plants are classified as edible, medicinal, building, hallucinogenic, or toxic. Knowing how to identify different types of plants can be a matter of life and death.

Before you go, make a "shopping" list of what is in season and what plant parts you intend to collect. The number of leaves, flowers, or fruit you eat can also be limited, so respect the dosage as advised in this book. Although medicinal plants may be beneficial for specific ailments, remember that just because one part of a plant is edible, not all aspects may be. For example, comfrey has leaves that can be applied to the skin but are not edible. Some plants, such as dandelions, can be used wholly for food or medicinal purposes. Flowers and leaves can be used to make tea or added to a salad, while the roasted roots are used as a substitute for coffee and are beneficial for many alignments used in folk medicine.

Your next step is to go foraging; check to see if the plant is endangered or poisonous. You should now be able to check off at least three of the identifying features listed in this book, so only collect a plant if one of the criteria is met.

HOW TO IDENTIFY PLANTS

You will learn to recognize plants in your local area quickly if you join a guided field tour with an experienced guide.

- Learn the poisonous ones first, so you know which ones to avoid.
- Carefully observe the plants in nature and compare them to the picture in the field guide or plant identification book.
- Take measurements of the leaf or stem width or the width of the flower head.
- Check as many of the identifying features listed as possible.
- Check the habitat closely. What other plants are growing nearby? These often tell you the type of soil the plant is growing in, whether it is shady or sunny.

There are more than 51,000 species of plants in the world, and more than half of them belong to just six plant families. Among them are asters, the mint family, the mustard family, the parsley family, the pea family, and grasses. Let's look at the general characteristics and distinguishing features of each family.

The Aster/Sunflower Family: Asteraceae

The sunflower is a common flower that everybody recognizes! It is part of a massive group of plants such as dandelion, black-eyed Susan, gumweed, and even daisies. This family also includes artichokes, marigolds, and chrysanthemums. Of course, like any family, some varieties will be taller or shorter or have different features, but there are enough standard features to make some generalizations. The

Asteraceae is one of the biggest and most important flowering plant families. It has more than 19,000 species, including 2,687 in the US and Canada.

The flower shape is a common feature. It is usually saucerlike or disc-shaped, and petals often radiate from a center. It may have colorful petals like sunflowers, asters, dandelions, and daisies, but sagebrush does not have these; having them is not essential.

A single flower is often a composite. This means that the flower head is not a single flower. If you examine it closely, you will see many tiny flowers in bunches. When you look at aster, dandelion, and sunflower heads, you will notice that sometimes there are multiple smaller flowers within one flower head. These are attached at a base, and each part produces a seed eventually. Think of how each tiny brown flower in the center of a sunflower head becomes a seed. In a dandelion, remember that each fluffy white part of the piece we blow contains a seed at the end of it!

Are there multiple bracts? A bract is a modified leaf that wraps around the flower bud, and this family often has one or even two layers of this outer layer. Think of a sunflower with the dried, brown, leafy parts surrounding the flower head. Artichoke buds also have bracts, which are pulled off and eaten when the fruit is ripe.

Example: dandelion(*Taraxacium officinale*) Diagram 1, (page 63)

The Mint Family: Lamiaceae

Well-known members of this family include catnip, pepper-mint, spearmint, basil, and marjoram. Think of the distinc-tive smell of these plants and identify this family.

There are approximately 3,500 plants in this family, and their identifying features are:

1. *Square stems.* The stem may look round when growing, but if you pick a piece of it, you will see the interior shape looks square and has four sides.
2. **Leaves grow directly opposite the stem.** Observe two leaves and see how one leaf grows left and the other grows directly opposite on the right-hand side of the stem. The following leaves do the same but spread on a different axis, which allows the leaves to gain maximum light. In other plant families, leaves grow on the left, have a gap, and more on the right or in circles around the stem.
3. **It smells of mint.** If any plant has a scent of mint, it is unmistakably mint. Rub a leaf in your hand to see if it releases a smell. The volatile aromatic oil from these plants is antimicrobial too. The leaves can be used in teas, and many are edible.

Example: self-heal (*Prunella vulgaris*) Diagram 2, page 64,

The Mustard Family: Brassicaceae

Mustard and watercress are often added to egg-based mayonnaise, and many of us are familiar with this family spread as a garnish on salad dishes. The leaf taste is a give-away; some are peppery and some have a tang, but you want to add just a few leaves to any dish because too many will overpower your tongue. Plants from the cabbage and water-cress families are also included in the mustard family. An important identifying feature of this family is the flower. Garlic mustard is a weed that has spread widely from Europe to the US. In some parts of the US, it has become a problem. It is a tasty leaf, full of vitamins, and a great addi-tion to a forager's bag since it is everywhere. There are approximately 3,200 plants in this family.

Example: shepherd's purse (*Capsella bursa-pastoris*) Diagram 4, page 66,

Their identifying features are:

1. The flowers have four petals, often in an X shape or a cross, and are often yellow, although there are whitish varieties too. Think of the bright yellow fields covered with rapeseed flowers in late spring.
2. Seeds grow in racemes. A raceme is a flower head with separate bunches of blooms that are attached to the main flower stem by thinner, short stems. These look like the spokes of the umbrella when you look closely! The seeds grow in spirals around the stem and come in different shapes. For example, garlic

mustard has long, pointed, oblong seed pods, which turn brown when ripe.

3. They will have two short stamens and four taller ones. A stamen is part of a flower that holds pollen; the bee fertilizes this when it visits the flower. In the mustard family, the size of the stamens is not the same.

The Parsley Family : Umbellifers or Apiaceae

Some members of this family include our well-known common vegetables and herbs like wild carrots, celery, cumin, anise, dill, and, obviously, parsley. But this family also consists of the most poisonous plants in the US, such as poison hemlock and water hemlock. Because this family's edible and medicinal plants look much like the more dangerous ones, it is imperative to tell them apart.

There are approximately 3,780 plants in this family, and their identifying features are:

1. The flowers have an identifiable umbrella-shaped flower, which can be white, creamy, or yellow-colored. This is called a *compound umbel*, and the width of this flower head varies enormously. It can be tiny (like the wild carrot flowers) or massive (like the Giant Hogweed). The flower head comprises many smaller flowers, which is the compound part of the description.

2. Hollow stalks are another identifying feature of this family. Think of a stick of celery, and you get the idea! These come in various colors, from green to pinkish-purple, and various width sizes. They may be smooth or hairy to the touch, but they are usually hollow when you cut the stem. But not all of them

3. The leaves may offer a clue, but this is not always the case, so use the two features above to identify them correctly. Parsley family members are mostly with alternate feather-like divided leaves that are sheathed at the base. Size are variable big as Cow parsnip and small even thread like herbs as dill (*Anethum graveolens*),and fennell (*Feoniculum*)

4. Remember the poisonous varieties! Some plants in this family look similar due to umbel flower heads, but they are toxic. Always wear gloves, and it is best not to touch any plant you fear may be poisonous.

Example: Cow parsnip (*Heracleum maximum*) Diagram 3 page 65,

The Pea Family: Fabaceae

There is a wide variety of plants, including sweetpeas, white and red clovers, mimosas, purple milkvetch, wild licorice, and peas. The mimosa flowers

do not have the exact flower description, but they have distinctive seed pods.

There are approximately 13,000 species worldwide, and their identifying features are:

- They have irregularly shaped flowers with five petals and the "banner, wings, and keel." These terms describe the formation of the petals in a pea flower. The banner is one single petal that looks as though two petals have been joined together. The wings are the next closest petals, which can expand outward or take various shapes. The keel petals are the last two and are usually joined together. Bees land on the keel and then enter the flower's interior. There are often multiple flowers.

- The seeds are in pods. Usually, the seeds look like peas in a pod and dry out to a brown color, often with pointed ends, which you need to break to release the seeds.

- Sometimes, these are climbers with tendrils. It is not true of all plants in this family, but if you think of peas, sweet peas, and climbing vines, they are often a clue.

- Leaves differ in different subfamilies. Some are Trifolium. This Latin translates as three leaves, which describes the cloverleaf perfectly! Others are compounds, with smaller leaves combining into one leaf. Pinnate leaves have smaller leaves spreading from a central point on the stem, like the fingers on your hand and your thumb, which all attach to a central point.

Example: red clover (*Trifolium pratense*) Diagram 5, page 67,

The Grass Family: Poaceae

There are more than 9,000 species of grass worldwide, and many have been bred specifically to make the grain crops we know today as cereals, such as oats, corn, wheat, barley, rice, and sorghum wheat. Mormon tea is a grass used to treat kidney alignment. Drinking tea made from its green growth can cause kidney and urinary tract infections. Plants that look like grass don't have woody stems. Instead, they have hollow, jointed stems wrapped in narrow leaves. Their flowers don't have petals, and their fruit looks like grain. Identify them by stem leaf shapes, nodes, seed shape, and position.

Example: Oat *(Avena sativa)* Diagram 6, page 68,

The best way to identify grasses is to look at the season, the landscape in which they are growing, and whether or not the seed head is visible. The height is another good indicator.

Now you can go on foraging trips with an expert and contribute important information about plant families. It's time to get your book packed in your rucksack with your tools, and let's move on to the next chapter, where we will examine the landscape of the Southwestern states and which medicinal plants you can expect to find there.

PLANTS DIAGRAMS

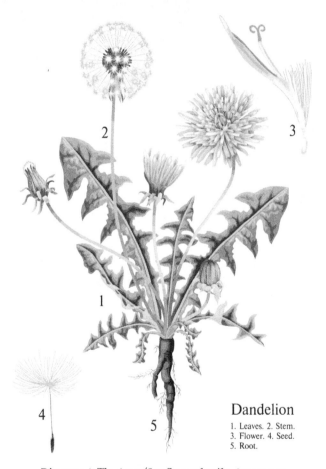

Dandelion
1. Leaves. 2. Stem.
3. Flower. 4. Seed.
5. Root.

Diagram 1: The Aster/Sunflower family-Asteraceae

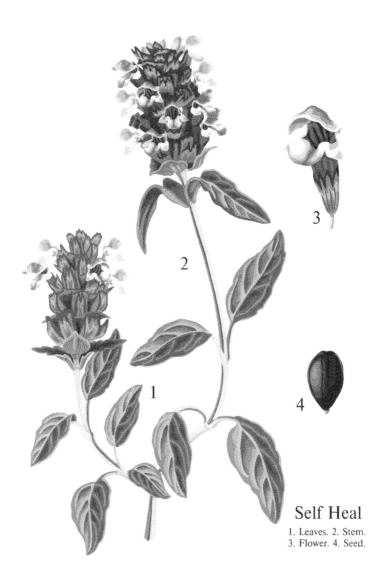

Self Heal

1. Leaves. 2. Stem.
3. Flower. 4. Seed.

Diagram 2: The Mint Family-Lamiaceae

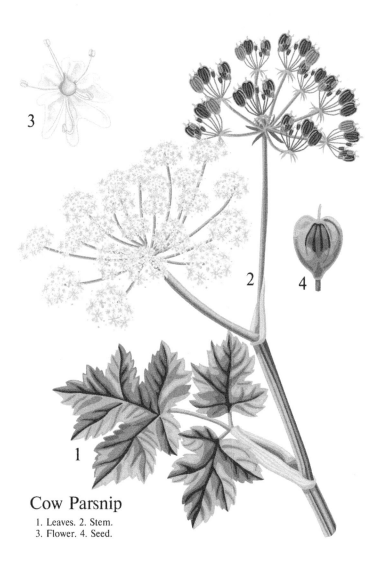

Cow Parsnip

1. Leaves. 2. Stem.
3. Flower. 4. Seed.

Diagram 3: The Parsley family- Umbellifers or Apiaceae.

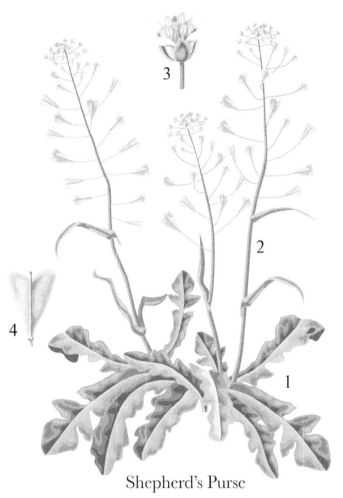

Shepherd's Purse

1. Leaves. 2. Stem.
3. Flower. 4. Seed.

Diagram 4: The Mustard family-Brassicaceae

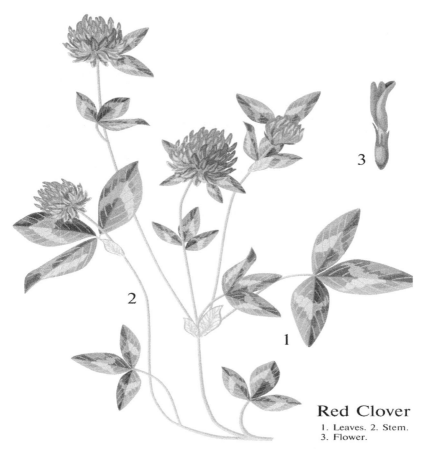

Red Clover

1. Leaves. 2. Stem.
3. Flower.

Diagram 5: The Pea family-Fabaceae (Leguminosae)

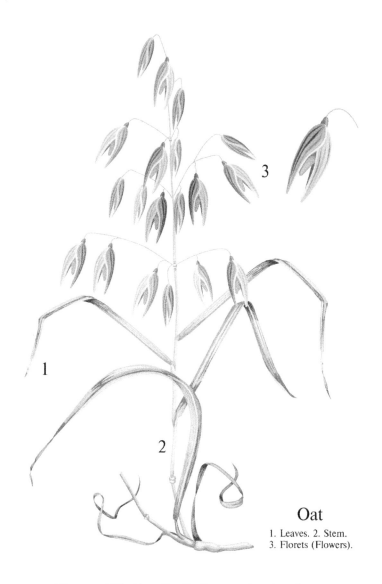

Oat

1. Leaves. 2. Stem.
3. Florets (Flowers).

Diagram 6: The Grass Family (Poaceae, Gramineae)

Making Sure These Skills Are Never Lost Again

"There is no wealth like knowledge, and no poverty like ignorance."

— BUDDHA

As you may recall from the introduction, the use of medicinal plants was, at one time, a skill passed down from generation to generation.

It's knowledge we should all have, but over time, we've lost touch with nature, and the essential skills we need to identify, collect, and make use of Earth's natural medicine cabinet are no longer being passed down.

But all is not lost. By sharing our knowledge now, we can stage an intervention and bring ourselves back to this fundamental understanding of the world – and when we do that, we'll have the skills to pass on to our own children.

The best part is, it's an easy job. You've already started by picking up this book and discovering the wonderful world of medicinal plants in Southwestern US.

And you can take it a step further – without even leaving your couch!

By leaving a review of this book on Amazon, you'll let other readers know where they can find this essential

guidance – and you'll be passing knowledge on just as our ancestors did.

Simply by letting other readers know how this book has helped you and what they'll find within its pages, you'll be guiding them towards this fundamental knowledge – and the benefits will be reaped generations down the line.

Thank you so much for your support. Together, we can rediscover nature's bounty and make sure the generations that come after us have everything they need to benefit from it.

Scan the QR code below to leave your review!

5

LAWS AND LANDS

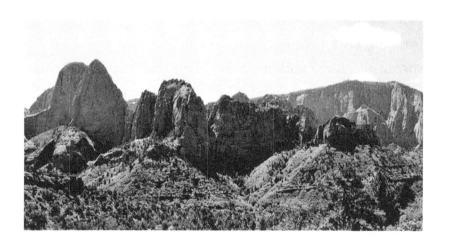

LEGAL ASPECTS OF FORAGING

This chapter examines the laws about picking wild plants in Arizona, California, Colorado, New Mexico, Nevada, Oklahoma, Texas, and Utah. This guide focuses on the medicinal plants found in these states. Let's start by discussing the laws in the US and these states. Then, we'll talk about the climate and environment in each state and the plants you can expect to find there. Look at Table 2. (page 88)

It may surprise you that many laws forbid us to pick plants in parks, tasty blackberries on a rural hedge, or even fruit overhanging a private garden in a city. There are strict foraging laws because plants are fragile, and pollution, the spread of cities, building work, construction, and farming are destroying their habitats. For wild plants on the endangered plant list, their very uncertain future and the fact that many species are being picked to death by over-eager foragers are frequently given as reasons you should not be free to harvest whatever, wherever. So, if you want to collect on private land, you should ensure you can do so before you go there. If it is a national park or a forested area, these are often federally owned with separate regulations for each state, which are covered below.

FORAGING LAWS AND NATIONAL PARKS

There are 59 national parks in the US, and there are many rules about foraging in public parks, forests, and federally owned land. Foraging in New York City parks is illegal, and there are cases of people being fined for picking dandelions or blackberries from Manhattan to Chicago.

Picking anything is restricted in California state parks, and regulation in Texas is strict. County park regulations vary, but almost all prohibit collecting plants, berries, leaves, stems, and any part of the plant. Like many other states, the Southwest region has regulations against the collection of mushrooms. You should know that many laws say that you can only collect wild plants for your own use and not sell them.

Most federally owned land, like national parks, is governed by laws like the Organic Act of 1916. This law says that the public can use national parks, reservations, and monuments to "conserve the scenery and natural history" and to have fun, keeping in mind that future generations will also want to enjoy them.

It says that these lands must be left "unimpaired," which has been interpreted as a ban on picking, with the idea that future generations should be able to enjoy these open spaces as they are. This act also established the NPS (National Park Service) to promote and regulate the use of forests throughout the US.

The most important thing to understand is that the legislation is not uniform across the US. Because the rules vary by state, you should contact the landowner whose land you intend to pick and make arrangements with them before you arrive. The landowner may use herbicides on their property, and you want to avoid over-picking plants like ginseng. The Convention on International Trade in Endangered Species of Wild Fauna and Flora (CITES, 1975) protects wild ginseng internationally and in the US. This treaty is in place everywhere.[1] It has been decimated in the US and worldwide, so the regulation against picking is sensible.

Regulations in our 59 National Parks

Thirteen parks don't let people pick plants, while 46 do, but only in certain situations. The superintendent of each park decides what food can be collected and how much can be taken. The guide to the park explains what qualifies as "wild foods." This often refers to berries, nuts, flowers, leaves, etc.

Some parks have specific areas where picking isn't allowed, and they have to say that foraging is only for personal use to stop people from taking plants to sell. Digging is not often permitted, so remember that if you are searching for roots. Some parks also ban tools, and you must only use your hands to forage. You should always stay in designated walking areas and not wander into forests or mountainous areas. Climbing trees is often prohibited, and you must only pick what you can from the ground.

Mushrooms, lobsters, and fiddlesticks can't be taken from 10 National Parks, but this varies from park to park. The collection of fish and algae in coastal areas is prohibited, as is the collection of antlers or nests. It is against the law to bring in new plants or animals, so you can't spread seeds you got somewhere else unless you are part of a forestry conservation group that is allowed to do so.

Be careful what tools you leave in your car, too, because restrictions are placed on possessing a mineral or metal detector, magnetometer, side-scan sonar, or sub-bottom profiler (unless you are in a boat in these areas).

Native American tribes and members enrolled in a tribe may not have to follow all of these rules. Check the agreed-upon collection sites set by federal law or regional treaties with individual tribes.

COLLECTION IN THE SOUTHWESTERN STATES

This section examines the medicinal plants you can harvest and where you can find them, state by state. For your convenience, at the end of this section is a table listing the environments found in each state and the typical plants growing there. Weather extremes in the Southwest range from heat waves to cold, droughts and floods, snow and blizzards in the high mountains, and arid desert areas with little rainfall.

Arizona

This state is usually called arid because it doesn't get much rain. For example, the deserts in southwestern Arizona only get about 8 cm (3 inches) of rain a year. Still, high mountains in the west have much more rainfall than the deserts, which causes different plants to thrive there. In southwest Arizona, the more elevated areas get between 25 and 30 inches (65-76cm) of rain each year, while the lower regions get less than 3 inches (8 cm).

The Grand Canyon, one of the world's seven wonders, was carved by the Colorado River and showed geological history in the formation of the ancient rocks. Most of it was formed below sea level, and we see it due to the uplift of the Colorado Plateau. Due to the uplift, the river's gradient became steeper, which increased the ability of the water to cut through the rock.

Arizona often has thunderstorms from July to September, which can be deadly, especially if lightning is predicted. Check the park website before you leave and plan to collect on another day if the weather forecast is for monsoonal thunderstorms. If you get caught out in a thunderstorm, take cover. Listen for thunder, watch for lightning, and remember that flash floods or falling rocks may occur during or after storms.

Can you collect medicinal plants in Arizona?

Plants listed as native or endangered by the Arizona Department of Agriculture cannot be picked, cut, dug up, or moved without permission. The website has a place to get a permit and a form to fill out if you want to remove a protected plant. They also have a list of protected native plants by category. The Arizona Revised Statutes (Title 3, Chapter 7, Arizona Native Plants) tell you which plants are protected and say that you need a license to get rid of any of these plants. Permits can be purchased in person at the Phoenix and Tucson offices. Native Plant Rules and the Arizona Department of Agriculture and Forestry, This Historical Note and New Section, recodified from 3 AAC 4, Article 6, at 10 AAR 726, go into effect on February 6, 2004 (Supp. 04-1).

California

California has deserts, coasts, mountains, and various plants to suit each environment. In this semi-tropical state with endless sunshine, there are many fruits, flowers, nuts, and plants to forage. Unfortunately, foraging is generally frowned upon, forbidden, and punished with hefty fines. Since California also has a coastline on the ocean, picking seaweed or other plants that grow in the water is strictly regulated and requires a permit based on the amount collected and the area. You can find seaweed and algae on beaches in Orange County, San Diego County, and Los

Angeles County, but you need the right paperwork. Coastal foraging has strict limits on quantities collected.

Nine national parks are included: Channel Island, Death Valley, Joshua Tree, Lassen Volcanic, Petrified Forest, Pinnacles, Redwood, Sequoia and Kings Canyon, and Yosemite. In state parks and forests, harvesting always requires a permit. This state prohibits collecting berries and wild foods. Foraging is restricted in California's national parks and the state, so always get permission before collecting.

Other considerations:

California is listed as hostile to foragers on various websites I have researched. This is because, in the past, private landowners passed laws that made it illegal for Native Americans, people who used to be slaves, and subsistence farmers to go on private land and pick berries, cacti, green leaves, and nuts.

Can you collect medicinal plants in California?

Even though it is usually against the law to take plants, Salt Point State Park lets people forage for mushrooms. The main reason foraging is restricted is the damage caused by crowds of people, who enable pathogens to invade trees and may also encourage people off the regulated trails.

If you wish to forage for medicinal plants in California, it is best to seek out private landowners and ask permission to harvest on their land. Private landowners can sell or donate plants that grow on their land, provided the plant is not on the endangered list.

Colorado

Colorado has a continental climate with low humidity. Temperatures, rainfall, and snowfall in this state vary greatly depending on where you are and the time of year. The eastern plains have hot (but windy) summers with frequent thunderstorms. The warmest temperatures in the Southwest are in Arizona and New Mexico, while Colorado and Utah are among the lowest[2]. In high mountains, like on the Colorado Plateau, temperatures decrease as you get higher. Estimate an approximately 3°F (1.5°C) decrease for each 1,000-foot (300 m) increase in mountain height and dress accordingly. Heavy snow falls in winter on the high mountains. Temperatures differ significantly between high mountains and lower areas. When comparing Pikes Peak at 14,114 feet (4302 meters), which is only 90 miles (145 km) away from Las Animas at 3898 feet (1188 meters), the temperature difference has been compared to the difference between chilly Iceland and sunny Florida.

Can you collect medicinal plants in Colorado?

Colorado's state and national parks don't allow people to look for food unless they are in a life-or-death situation and need to eat. Seventeen plants in Colorado are currently federally listed as threatened or endangered, so none can be touched. The Colorado Rare Plant Conservation Strategy aims to protect the most endangered plant species in Colorado and the places where they live. The strategy has been developed by the Colorado Rare Plant Conservation Initiative (RPCI), a diverse partnership of state and federal agencies, private organizations, academic institutions, and individuals concerned with the stewardship of habitat and plants in Colorado[3]. Proactive conservation actions aim to avoid population declines, conserve habitats, and generate publicity to make the public aware of Colorado's endangered plant species.

A part of this document states that valuable medicines come from native plants, e.g., the West's Pacific yew (*Taxus brevifolia*) contains taxol, a powerful cancer treatment, and Colorado's heartleaf arnica (*Arnica cordifolia*) is used to treat sprains and bruises. Colorado intends to conserve its plant heritage and advise people about its collection[4].

Two different cabinet-level agencies administer state parks and forested areas. In addition to the NPS (the US Forest Service), which resides within the Department of Agriculture, there are National Forest units. The Forest Service may have different rules about foraging in the national forests it manages than the NPS. You will need to check with both before you start collecting.

Location is also crucial. Even though NPS rules usually don't require permits, someone who wanted to go foraging in a national forest would first have to read the Forest Service's complicated and detailed fee and permit schedule for "harvesting special forest products" in the park. The forest's rules also include requirements for permitting, age, location, quantity, and other variables.

Nevada

Nevada is a dry state with hot and sticky summers and short, harsh winters with lots of snow and strong winds. It is a mountainous region with semi-arid grasslands and a sandy, alkaline desert. The temperature generally ranges from 26° to 90°F (-3° to 32°C).

As a forager, the critical fact about Nevada is that nearly 80% of the land is managed by institutions such as the US Forest Service or the National Park Service (NPS).

There are specific rules regarding permissible quantities, locations, and other factors. You need to consult the permit schedule published by the forest and then purchase a permit to "harvest special forest products" and pay a fee. Eastern Mojave low ranges are in Arizona, California, Nevada, and Utah. See Arizona for more details.

Nevada has the Great Basin, Death Valley (only 3% of which is in Nevada), Lake Mead Park, Tule Springs Fossil Beds, Gold Butte, Basin and Range National Monument, and Spring Mountain National Recreation Area. There are also 12 state parks in the state. The plants of Nevada are based on desert plants such as mesquite, yuccas, cacti, sagebrush, and tumbleweeds.

Spring greens and various wildflowers thrive in the basins and elevations in the middle and offer foragers, currants, pinyon trees, and manzanita. Higher than this, there are wild roses, raspberries, and yampah. This changing landscape is a forager's heaven!

Can you collect medicinal plants in Nevada?

Like other states in the Southwest, Nevada's Department of Agriculture has a series of leaflets about noxious weeds and endangered species. Some rules allow foragers to harvest specific crops (e.g., pine nuts) from sites run by the Bureau of Land Management (BLM) and the Humboldt-Toiyabe National Forest. There are limits to the quantities in which you can pick them. Without a permit, foragers can harvest up to 25 pounds of the nuts per year for personal use, not for resale.

New Mexico

New Mexico has an arid, semi-arid, or continental climate, which means it gets little rain and humidity and has a lot of bright sunshine. Like all the southwestern states, there is a lack of moisture in the air, and daytime heat dissipates quickly at dusk. However, the temperature difference between night and day is not as extreme as in Arizona; here, it ranges from 25° to 35°F (14° to 19°C). New Mexico tends to have dry winters because the rainfall coming from the Pacific falls on the mountains in Arizona and Utah, leaving very little by the time it reaches New Mexico. Summer rainfall on the Great Plains comes in intense thunderstorms. The annual rainfall is less than 10 inches (25 cm) on the Great Plains and Basin, but range regions get more than 20 inches (50 cm) in the higher mountainous areas of the northwestern part of the state. Summer rains fall almost entirely during brief but intense thunderstorms on the Great Plains, although the occasional hurricane in the Gulf of Mexico may push heavier rainfall inland[5].

There are two national parks, Carlsbad Caverns and White Sands, two national historic parks, Chaco Culture and Pecos, and one national heritage area, the Northern Rio Grande.

Can you collect medicinal plants in New Mexico?

The Bureau of Land Management (BLM) manages the parks. You need a permit from the BLM to collect medicinal plants, and you can only use the plants for yourself.

With this permit, you can collect limited amounts (up to 5 gallons) of berries, nuts, and cones in addition to 25 pounds of greenery or boughs *per species*. Twenty-five pounds of pinyon nuts are allowed per household. Other charges apply for trees, shrubs, etc. There are also treaties with local Native American tribes that give them the right to pick plants as part of their traditions. Before you go to private land, you must contact the owner.

Oklahoma

Texas borders Oklahoma to the west and south and New Mexico to the west. It sits partly in the Great Plains, known as America's breadbasket, and features parts of the Cross Timbers region and the US Interior Highlands. Oklahoma has many environments, including mountain ranges, prairies, grasslands, mesas, and forests.

This state is in a humid subtropical region, a transitional climate zone in the US. Oklahoma is known for severe weather, mainly encompassing the region known as Tornado Valley. It sits between three contrasting air currents, resulting in destructive storms. This area is prone to tornadoes, thunderstorms, high winds, and big hail. Weather and temperatures can change rapidly in short periods of time. Oklahoma is warmer and wetter in the east than in the west. In general, the temperature ranges between 100 °F and 0 °F (38 °C and 18 °C), but it can get hotter or colder in certain parts of the state.

Can you collect medicinal plants in Oklahoma?

Oklahoma has a rich Native American heritage; many still forage for food. It means that it's generally a forager-friendly state. You should still double-check and ask for permission on private land.

Texas

Texas is the second-largest state in the United States. It borders Oklahoma and New Mexico. Most people think this state is mostly desert, but it also has prairies, grasslands, forests, and coastlines. You can also find swampland, plains, hills, and mountains in the expansive territory. Alaska has a larger area, and California has more people.

Texas is large enough to have multiple climate zones with variable weather. While it's associated with hot, airy deserts, large parts of Texas are subtropical and humid. Generally, you will find wetter climates to the east of Texas and more arid climates to the west. Texas is prone to storms, flooding, and tornadoes. Depending on where you are in Texas, you can experience temperatures below freezing on winter nights and temperatures that peak in the 90s during summer.

Can you collect medicinal plants in Texas?

Most state and federal lands in Texas don't allow people to pick plants unless they need to for survival. If foraging on private property, ask permission, as foraging without permission is considered stealing.

Utah

This state offers high mountain ranges in the north and west, which shelter the rest of the state from either heavy rainfall or snowfall. Heavy snowfall can be found in these high mountainous areas, such as the Sierra Nevada and the Cascade mountains, but these high elevations shade the rest of the state from freezing temperatures and cold. Utah is far from the Gulf of Mexico and the Pacific, meaning less rainfall and a warm, sunny climate. Rain travels eastward over the mountains; by the time it reaches the rest of the state, little is left to fall. This state is proud of its five national parks: Arches, Bryce Canyon, Canyonlands, Capitol Reef, and Zion.

Foraging environments such as red rock deserts and alpine meadows are available to the forager, and the contrast between these environments explains the variety of plants available for foraging. The eastern Mojave lowlands are in Arizona, California, Nevada, and Utah.

The native plants range from unique trees such as the bristlecone pine to flowering penstemons, which come in 100 slightly different varieties in Utah. Native American tribes have used red penstemon (internally and externally) for its analgesic qualities. It was also used to ease stomach aches and period pain. The Goshute, Navajo, Piute, Shosne, and Ute people inhabited parts of Utah, and their knowledge of plants is being shared and published. If you search alphabetically, the medicinal uses of these plants are discussed in detail in Part ll.

Can you collect medicinal plants in Utah?

Collecting medicinal plants in Utah can only be done if you purchase a permit from the BLM and the material is for personal use.

With this permit, you can collect limited amounts (up to 5 gallons) of berries, nuts, and cones in addition to 25 pounds of greenery or boughs per species. Twenty-five pounds of pinyon nuts are allowed per household. Less than ten trees, less than 20 shrubs, cacti, or grass are considered for personal use. Additional charges apply to trees at $2 per foot or a minimum of $10 per tree. Shrubs and cacti are two each, and grasses and wildflowers are $1 each.

Other essential details.

- You must buy a permit to transplant a shrub, bulb, or tree.
- You must drive on existing roads, and no vehicle is permitted to leave the road, so all collection must be done on foot.
- Collecting plant or tree material from wilderness study areas is not permitted. Check this when you buy your permit, and show them where you intend to pick.

In Chapter 6, we'll talk about different ways to go foraging so that you can find and use medicinal plants safely.

TABLE 2: A SUMMARY OF WHAT YOU CAN EXPECT TO HARVEST, STATE BY STATE

State	Environment type	Plants you will find
Arizona	Desert: arid e,g. The Sonoran Desert	brittlebush, cottonwood, cocklebur, cacti, and succulents; jojoba, mesquite, ironwood, palo verde, and saguaro.
	Eastern Mojave woodland and low ranges - arid This area borders Utah, California, and Nevada.	Blackberry, Buttonbush, Cat's Claw, Creosote Bush, Juniper, Hoptree, Horsetail, Gumtree, Mesquite, Oak, Ocotillo, Passion Flower, Pine (pinyonPinyon), Silk Tassel, Wild Rose and Rosehips, Wild Lettuce, Willows, and Yucca.
	Low valleys Lower Grand Canyon – desert scrub.	Acacia, Amaranth, Arrowweed, Asparagus, Burdock, Brittle Bush, California Bay Laurel, Cat's Claw, Cottonwood, Creosote Bush, Desert Verbena, Gumtree, Mesquite, Ocotillo, Tamarisk, and Willows.
California	Desert	Agave, Barrel Cactus, Cholla, Creosote Bush, Desert Verbena, Joshua Tree, Ocotillo, Prickly Pear Cactus, Saguaro.
	Coastal, and meadows	California poppy, Mullein, Passion flower, Salvia, Western Peony, Desert Verbena.
	Mojave Basin and range.	Acacia, Agave, Creosote Bush, Coyote Willow, Desert Willow, Galleta Grass, Joshua Trees, Mesquite, Smoke tree, White bursage.
Colorado	Grand Canyon and desert Colorado Desert (a northern arm of the Sonoran desert), which is lower, hotter, and drier.	Creosote bush, California Prickly Pear cactus, Desert sand verbena,
	Mountain Rockies – Deep snow in winter. Above 3000 feet	Heartleaf Arnica, Banana yucca, Bergamot, Dandelion, Cattails, Fantails, wild Strawberries and Asparagus, Wild onion, Orache, Salsify, Mustard, Prickly lettuce, Pine, Wild asparagus, wild plums.
	Desert – big drop between day and night temperatures	*Asclepius*, Cocklebur, Copperleaf, Cow parsnip, Cudweed, Fanpetals, Prickly Pear Cactus.

| Nevada | Basin

Nevada's flora is of desert orientation, its division by ribbons of transition-mountain-s ubalpine-alpine plant life is an important aspect. | Amaranth, Beeplant, Biscuitroot, Bitterroot, Cattail, Checkermallow, Chia, Chokecherry, Creeping Hollygrape, Currant, Elder, Evening Primrose, Field Pennycress, Gooseberry, Ground Cherry, Hollygrape, Lambsquarters, Lemonade Berry, Manzanita, Maple, Mariposa Lily, Mesquite, Miner's Lettuce, Monkey Flower, Mullein, Nettle, Oak, Pine, Plantain, Raspberry, Thistle, Tumble Mustard, Tumbleweed, Watercress, Wild Onion, Wild Rose, Wild Sunflower, Wintercress,Yampah, Yellow dock, Yucca |
|---|---|---|
| | Mountain –subalpine and alpine | Wild roses, raspberries, and yams grow alongside aspen and fir trees. Currant, Hop Bush, Pine (pinyon), and Manzanita. |
| | Basin | Anemone, Horseweed, Hound's Tongue, Mimosa |
| | Desert | Prickly pear, Yucca, barrell Cactus, Desert anemone, |
| New Mexico | Desert | Bearberry, sometimes Bloodberry, Black-eyed Susan, Buffalo Gourd, Butterfly Weed, Cotton Leaf, Desert Sand Verbena, Jimson, Lobelia, Mugwort, Wild Mustard, Sunflower, and Yucca. |
| | Mountains | Anemone, Apache Plume, Bee Balm, Black-eyed Susan, Cattail, Chickweed, Chokecherry, Currant, Dandelion, Devil's Claw, Gooseberry, Juniper, Lobelia, Lambsquarters, Mallow, Manzanita, Marsh Marigold, Mesquite, Mormon tea, Mullein, Nettle, Oak, Pinyon Pine, Prickly Pear, Purslane, Raspberry, Sumac, Thistle, Tuber Starwort, Tule, Tumble Mustard, Watercress, Wild Grape, Wild Onion, Wild Rose, Wild Strawberry, Wild Sunflower, Wolfberry, Yellow Dock. |
| | Great Plains

Rapid thunderstorms bring rainfall in summer; drier winters. | Common Mallow, Dandelion, Dock, Echinacea (Purple Coneflower), Evening Primrose, Spanish needle, Sunflower, Wild tobacco, Yarrow, |

Texas	Northern Plains: semi-arid and prone to drought.	Prickly pear, Lemon bee balm, Horsetails, Horseweed, Plantain, Yarrow
	South Texas: Semi-arid and wetter valleys. The southernmost tip of the Great Plains region. Hot, humid summers and subtropical forest areas.	Ephedra, Filaree, Prickly pear, Purple sage, balloon vines, Lemon bee balm, Horsetails, Horseweed, Pimpernels, Plantain, Prickly ash, Yarrow
	Trans-Pecos Region (west): Deserts and mountains. Arid climate, with more wet and temperate climates in the mountainous areas.	Agarita, Agave, Cholla cactus, Desert willow, Ephedra, Prickly pear, Purple sage, Chaste tree, Cudweed, lemon bee balm, Horsetails, Horseweed, Mullein, Ocotillo, Plantain, Prickly ash, Yarrow
	Piney Woods (east): Humid subtropical. Coastal sections are prone to storms.	Prickly pear, Boneset, Carolina geranium, Chaste tree, Clover, Cudweed, Elderberry, Heal's all, Lemon bee balm, Horsetails, Lizard's tail, Mullein, Plantain, Prickly ash, Evening primrose, Fireweed, Yarrow
	Hill Country (central): Rivers and hills, semi-arid and sub-humid areas.	Prickly pear, Cucumber seed, Cudweed, Horehound, Lemon bee balm, Horsetails, Horseweed, Mullein, Pimpernel, Plantain, Prickly ash, Purple sage, Milk thistle, Yarrow

Utah	Southeast	Chickweed, Chokecherry, Currants, Gooseberries, Juniper, Mormon tea, Pinyon (pine), Prickly Pear Cactus, Prickly lettuce, Sow thistle, Stinging nettle, Strawberries, Raspberries, and Sumac.
	Meadow and Grassland.	Butterfly weed, Chickweed, Crane's bill, Sow thistle, Mormon tea, Prickly lettuce, Wild tobacco, and Stinging nettle.
Oklahoma	Mountains and plains	Bergamont, Pleurisy root, Goldenrod, Passion flower, Yarrow, Broomweed, Horsemint, Echinacea, Mullein, Spiderwort, Plantain, carolina geranium, Evening primrose, Rough leaf dogwood, Purple poppy mallow, Elderberry, Ironweed, Horsemint

FORAGING TECHNIQUES

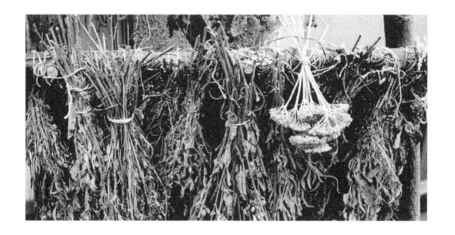

HARVESTING ESSENTIALS

The first and most important thing to learn about harvesting plants is to always identify the species correctly and with certainty. Only harvest something when you're 100% sure of what it is. This means making sure that the plant's growth cycle matches the time of year that the species usually grows. Once you know what the plant is, you should ensure that it is healthy. The leaves, flowers, roots, and seeds alike should be healthy. There should be no discoloration to speak of. Avoid any plants with blackened or moldy parts. However, some insect damage is acceptable, as you will never find a perfect specimen in the wild. When you've established that the plant is healthy and that it's the right time to forage it, you can harvest the parts of the plant that you need.

When harvesting the leaves and other plant parts, only take what you need. Leave enough to allow future growth. Most plants have leaves and stems that branch off the main stem. You should take the top third of the leaves; these are generally better. Pinch them off just above the leaf nodes, where new growth occurs. You're bruising the leaf as little as possible when you pinch off leaves, especially if they're delicate

herbs. If the plant doesn't branch out but grows on a single stem, cut the top third to two-thirds off and leave the rest to allow it to regrow. If you're harvesting stems, use a sharp cutting tool and aim just above a node. Keep the spines in mind when gathering cactus pads. Wear long sleeves and thick gloves, and use tongs to grasp the pad while you cut it away from where it joins another pad. Store in a burlap or fabric bag, then scrape off the spines at home.

Flowers and flower parts are commonly used for food and medicine. You can harvest them as buds, but the best time to harvest medicinal flowers is on dry mornings, just before they are fully open. This ensures that they have as many oils in them as possible. If the flowers grow in clusters, like yarrow or elderflowers, remove the whole stem for ease and retrieve the flowers later. Otherwise, use a cutting tool to snip off the flower heads.

While we may think of fruits as soft, edible berries or larger fruit, botanically, the word "fruit" refers to the seed-carrying structure left behind after flowers die. If you're dealing with soft fruit, gently pull them away with your fingers. Never try to forcibly remove fruit; if it doesn't come out easily, it's likely underripe. Fruit is designed to fall away when ripe. Some fruit can be harvested from the ground after falling, but check for damage. Nuts are also a kind of fruit. They're usually still in their husks when gathered, so you will have to pick them up off the ground and remove the husks and shells later. If the nuts are bitter, you can reach them by grinding them, then letting them soak in cold water to remove excess tannins. Soak them for 24 hours, refresh the water, and soak them for another 24 hours. Repeat until the bitterness is gone. Some plants, like poppies, leave behind seed pods or heads rather than produce fruit. You can simply place a bag over the ripe seed pod and shake it to collect the seeds. Otherwise, cut the stem underneath the seed pod and hang it upside down somewhere in your house to let the seeds fall naturally.

You should harvest the bark of most trees and shrubs in the spring because the bark peels away more easily. Some evergreens and conifers can be harvested year-round, however. Harvest bark from specimens at least 3-5 years old for the best results. Never remove bark directly from the tree trunk, but cut off a branch and strip the

bark from there. The inner bark is used for medicine, as this is where the plant's vascular system is found. Remove the outer bark first, then peel away the softer inner bark.

It's usually best to harvest roots in the spring or fall. When harvested in the fall, the roots of plants that have lived for two years or longer have more nutrients, sugars, and medicinal components. However, spring roots are often sweeter. The method for harvesting roots depends on the type of root. Tap roots are long and thick and must be carefully dug out with a sharp spade (Hori Hori) so that you can remove the root intact. When harvesting fibrous roots, you can dig around the plant and uproot it, but there are only so many plants in the area. Root harvesting is more destructive than other plant parts, so only take what you need. If you can cut off a section of the root without harming the plant too much, do so. Digging down 3–4 inches from the plant is usually possible. Once the root is removed, bang it against the ground to remove loose dirt and wash it before use. You may need to scrub or even peel the root before using it.

IMPROVING YOUR FORAGING TECHNIQUE

Many edible and medicinal plants can't be grown on farms, so they can only be found in the wild. Of course, it doesn't mean that they should be overlooked, which is where foraging comes into the picture. By getting better at foraging, you can get more plants, get better ones, and make sure that the plant can continue to grow without hurting the environment.

As mentioned in previous chapters, you should always be aware of local foraging laws. Private lands are a good option, as you can get permission from the landowners. This also means that you might be a sole forager, which reduces the risk of over foraging in an area. Pay attention to the soil quality and any nearby agricultural or industrial areas. If there is nearby water, then make sure it's unpolluted. Around these places, the land may still have chemicals, pathogens, herbicides, or heavy metals that plants can take in.

When harvesting, you should always aim to be sustainable and progressive. This means you're considering the plants, the local wildlife, and other harvesters. Even if a plant seems abundant in one area, it may not be abundant everywhere. Sustainable harvesting aims to reduce the damage you do, but progressive harvesting is the next step. A progressive forager will give back to the land while they are harvesting. They will spread seeds, remove invasive species, reintroduce native or helpful plants, and try to have as little effect as possible on the ecosystem. This also ties into the previous point about choosing good foraging locations. Don't wander too far off the beaten track and into the wilderness, as you may disturb local plant and animal life.

A responsible forager will only harvest a plant that they can reliably identify. This is one of those points that is worth repeating because it's so important. Some edible or beneficial plants have lookalikes with some of the same characteristics. It is possible to mistake a toxic plant for an edible one, which can have severe consequences. Take your time and learn about the parts of the plants you want to grow so you can tell them apart from others that look similar.

MEDICINAL PLANT PREPARATION TECHNIQUES

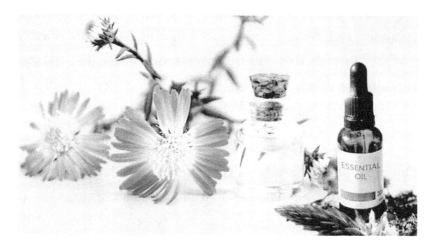

Once you've successfully harvested the medicinal plants, you must process them further to get the best results. Here is a breakdown of what you need to do when you bring your foraged plants home and how you can prepare and store them for later use.

CLEANING WILD PLANTS

No matter what you harvest, where you get it from, or how you plan on preparing your foraged plants, you will need to clean them. Dirt, insects, and other debris can and will find their way onto the plants. Harvesting is the first step to ensuring that wild edibles are clean. Always make sure you know what kind of plant it is and don't pick it near roads or places that may have been sprayed with chemicals. If you can, pick healthy, whole plants. This will reduce the chance that they will go bad and make them easier to clean. Brush off excess dirt in the field if you need to.

After bringing the wild plants home, place them in a colander and rinse them under running water to remove surface dust and any loose insects or debris. Fill a large container halfway with water and stir it occasionally. It dislodges dirt and insects. The herbs should float to the top of the water.

Once the plants have been rinsed and soaked, they must be dried. Because plants absorb water, a salad spinner is an excellent tool for removing excess water. To remove the majority of the water, you may need to use the spinner repeatedly, draining it between spins. After the excess water has been removed, the plants can be air dried.

Spread them out onto a towel to dry for as long as you need to; it depends on how you plan on using them. If you wish to use them fresh, leave them there for up to an hour or until the water evaporates. If you plan on using them for something else, such as an infusion, let them air dry for 24 hours. It will also remove some of their natural moisture, causing them to wilt.

STORING WILD GREENS

Wild greens, whether you plan to use them as food or medicine, can wilt quickly if they aren't stored properly. Here are some essential tips to ensure the best results:

Start early. Harvest greens in the morning before the sun has had a chance to dry them out.

When out and about, keep the greens in paper bags or breathable containers, and be sure not to overfill them.

Refresh greens in cold water to clean them and give them a new lease on life, following the earlier method.

Plastic retains heat. If you put foraged greens in plastic containers, they may wilt or go bad because of the extra heat.

Flowers and delicate greens can be easily crushed. It's best to store them in small containers. Use large leaves, such as nasturtium and burdock, as a buffer between layers of delicate plant parts. Damp paper towels can also work.

Refrigerate the greens as soon as possible. Keep them in a bag with a paper towel to absorb moisture.

Some tougher greens benefit from being blanched. Blanching preserves color while allowing you to store them for longer. You may need to blanch some plants before dehydrating or freezing them. After you've washed your greens, put them in a pot of boiling water for 10–20 seconds. Then immediately plunge them into a bowl of cold, preferably icy, water. This shocks the greens and stops the cooking process. From this point on, store and use as normal.

DRYING

People use dried herbs and food all the time, often for cooking or in tea blends. However, dried plants also carry much of the same medicinal value as fresh plants. Because dehydrating plants makes them much easier to store, you can use them for medicinal purposes all year. You can find dried herbs and flowers in stores, but you never know exactly how they were harvested or dried. Also, you can't find a different variety in the store than you can in the wild.

The first step in drying plants is the preparation phase. First, clean the plants. Pluck them from the stems if you're preparing delicate plant parts. When preparing tough plant parts such as roots, bark, or stalks, cut them into small pieces, ideally less than 14 inches thick. This ensures that they will dry all the way through and reduce drying time. Different drying methods also suit different plant parts better. Plant parts that are easy to break dry well on drying racks, in paper bags, and in a dehydrator. But woodier parts of the plant, like the roots, bark, stalks, and seeds, can be more efficiently dried using the oven, drying racks, the dehydrator, or hanging drying.

These are the different drying methods and how to achieve them:

A drying rack is an array of shelves stacked on top of each other with enough room for air to flow freely. You can buy them or even make them. Indoor racks should be placed somewhere clean that gets plenty of airflow. Somewhere near a sunny window is ideal, and you can cover the plants with cheesecloth if you're worried about dust. If it's dry, warm, and sunny, then feel free to put the drying rack outside. Avoid direct sunlight, as they can lose some of their colors, and bring them in if it's wet.

Hang-drying is a simple method for drying herbs. Keep them on the stalks and bundle them up, tying them at the bottoms of their stalks or stems with twine or bands. Hang the bundle upside down in an airy place until they're wilted or crunchy. This may take around two weeks.

If you want to dry delicate herbs on the go quickly, simply put them in a paper bag. Don't put too many wet herbs in the bag; leave it cracked open to allow moisture to escape. Place the paper bag somewhere hot and sunny, such as your car's dashboard or a windowsill.

The oven is best used for hardier plant parts, but you can use it to dry more delicate plants if you're careful. First, do the prep work mentioned earlier. Then lay out your harvest on a flat metal tray, like a cookie sheet, and put your oven on its lowest setting. Usually, this is about 120°F. Leave the oven door open to allow some heat to escape. Keep a close eye on them as they dry.

This method can take between 30 minutes and 3 hours, or even longer.

If you have a dehydrator, then you have a fantastic tool for drying plant parts. Generally, you want to dry delicate plant parts at lower temperatures, like 90°F, and tougher ones at closer to 120°F. Lay the prepared plant parts out on the dehydrator trays and follow the instructions on your dehydrator. It can take between 1-4 hours for leaves and 6–10 hours for roots or other hardy plant parts. Again, keep an eye on them and move the trays around periodically.

No matter what method you've used to dehydrate your plants, you must store them correctly to ensure they last as long as possible. Once the plant parts are dehydrated and brittle (delicate leaves should crumble), let them cool down. Put them into an airtight container, preferably made of glass. Then store them in a cool, dark place. They should last for about a year, but you can freeze them for more extended storage.

TEAS

Most commercial tea blends that people are familiar with contain leaves from the tea plant. However, you can make all kinds of other tea blends using the many plants that nature provides, which allows you to benefit from various health benefits and some genuinely delicious beverages.

You can use different preparation methods when making tea. Typically, your choice will depend on how many herbs you choose to use in your tea, whether you want to apply heat, and, if so, to what degree. You should also consider what, if anything, you plan to add to the tea, whether it's a mixer, water, or a sweetener of some kind. Always remember that the stronger the tea, the more you break up the herbs. Here are the three primary tea preparation methods:

Boiling plant parts in water is a quick and straightforward way to make tea. Most delicate herbs, like leaves and flowers, only need to be cooked for a few minutes before the flavors and aromas are released into the water. More challenging plant parts, like sassafras or dandelion roots, should be cooked for 15 to 30 minutes. Once the tea is boiled, the liquid should be poured through a strainer to remove any solid pieces. Cooking tea like this can destroy some plants' nutritional properties and isn't necessary for delicate, leafy plant parts. These can be steeped instead. If you want to keep the liquid (known as a decoction) for longer, it will keep in the refrigerator. Steeped tea is a great way to add herbal parts to hot water without losing any of the herbs' health benefits, as it is much gentler than boiling. Simply boil the water first and let the herbs sit in hot water for a few minutes to half an hour. There should be between two and four times more water than herbs by volume per serving. Once the herbs have steeped long enough, strain the tea into a cup and enjoy.

Making cold-infused tea is an even gentler way to infuse water with flavors, aromas, and beneficial components. This also produces a milder tea without the unpleasant bitterness from cooking the herbs. Most flowers and some fruits work best when infused this way. Simply put the herbs in a cold water container and refrigerate for a few hours or even a week. You can also leave it at room temperature, but keep an eye out for mold after two days. You can also infuse boiled or steeped tea to make it stronger by refrigerating the herbs in the liquid.

USE OF HERBAL PREPARATIONS

Now that we've explored different herbal teas, it's time to move on to other ways of preparing medical herbs. This is where tinctures, glycerites, and other herbal preparations come into play.

When creating a concentrated herbal preparation, such as a tincture, you should keep it in a dropper bottle. It makes it easier to store your herbal medication and administer accurate doses. Many of these herbal medicines have doses in milliliters, which means that being able to use drops ensures that you don't take too much of a particular medication. When using these dropper bottles, always transfer the medicine from the dropper to a spoon or cup before taking it. Do not take it directly from the dropper itself.

When taking herbal medicines, you should always research what you're taking to ensure it's safe. If you take any medications or have allergies, consult a doctor. And, as usual, only ever ingest something you've correctly and reliably identified.

Now we'll look into some other ways to prepare herbal medications.

Tinctures

A tincture can use plant parts, typically in combination with alcohol or vinegar, to draw out the plant's medicinal properties. Tinctures are known as herbal extracts, and you can also use them to concentrate the aroma or flavor of plants. Vanilla extract is often used in cooking, and other extracts of herbs are often used to make soap. When used medicinally, tincture dosages are typically between 2-4 mL, taken up to 3 times a day. They also take around 6–8 weeks to make but can be stored for years.

Alcohol is often the best medium to extract the beneficial components from plants (although there are some exceptions, such as nettle or raspberry leaves). Most people use strong white spirits, ideally at least 80 proof (40%). Don't go for anything too expensive; the taste isn't important. When making an alcoholic tincture, combine 1 part fresh herbs with 2 parts alcohol. If you're using dried herbs and roots, the ratio should be 1 part dried herbs to 5 parts alcohol. Allow it to sit for 6 to 8 weeks.

If you'd rather not use alcohol, you can use apple cider vinegar instead. The ratio remains the same. Stinging nettles also work better with vinegar, as it draws out their medicinal properties. Vinegar isn't as effective as alcohol, and these tinctures must be refrigerated. Still, they are more appropriate for children or people who prefer not to drink alcohol in any quantity. You can also use them in cooking.

Glycerite Tinctures

This tincture is similar to an alcohol or vinegar-based tincture but uses vegetable glycerine as a medium.

Glycerine is naturally sweet, which makes the tincture far more palatable than other mediums. It doesn't extract medicinal components as efficiently as alcohol and needs

refrigerated. The standard daily dose for a glycerite tincture is 1 ml, taken three times a day. Remember to drop the tincture onto a spoon and not take it directly from the stopper, as glycerine can get easily contaminated.

Oxymels

Oxymel is an ancient form of herbal medicine still used today. In their most basic form, oxymels are made up of apple cider vinegar and honey. The most common ratio is equal parts of both, but you can add more vinegar to make it sweeter. Then you can get the health benefits of both vinegar and honey in a way that tastes pretty good. If you've made a vinegar tincture, combine it with an equal amount of honey to create a medicinal oxymel. Take the oxymel as it is, or add it to a cup of boiled water for a quick honey tea. You can even use it in salad dressings.

Capsules

Herbal capsules are an easy way to take herbal medicines and make sure you get the right amount every time. It requires specialized equipment, but once you're set up, you can easily make as many as you like. You will need:

- Dehydrator
- High-powered blender or grinder
- Capsule machine
- Empty capsules
- Glass jars (for storage)

Once you have the equipment, the process is simple. Make sure you consult the instructions on your capsule machine.

1. Dehydrate your chosen herb or herbs, then blitz them to create a fine powder.
2. Set up the capsule machine base and halve the empty capsules. Put the longer halves in the slots of the capsule machine's base and the shorter halves on the top of the capsule machine.
3. Fill the capsules with the powder, ensuring it's evenly distributed. Fill the lower capsule halves.
4. Close the capsule machine, sealing the capsules. Then, place the finished capsules into the glass jar for storage.

Liniments

Liniments are used to relieve sore muscles and joints and treat circulation problems. Like a tincture, a liniment is just an essential oil or herb that has been steeped in a medium (like alcohol) that draws out the healing properties. The difference is that the liniment isn't ingested but is rubbed onto your skin. Here is a basic recipe that you can use.

Basic Herbal Liniment[1]

Ingredients:

- Rubbing alcohol, vodka, or witch hazel extract
- Fresh or dried herbs, bark, or flower (see notes)
- Optional: menthol crystals and essential oil

Method:

1. Select your herbs or plant parts. What you use depends on what you want to treat with the liniment. Clean the plant parts if needed, then roughly chop them into approximately ½-inch pieces.
2. Put the chopped fresh herbs or dried herbs into a clean glass jar. Cover them with alcohol.
3. Seal the jar and leave it for around six weeks. Shake it once a day.
4. Strain out the herbs and return the liniment to the jar. Rub a small amount onto your skin when needed.

Notes:

Spices and herbs like cayenne, rosemary, black pepper, and ginger can help with poor circulation.

Cottonwood or aspen buds and bark can help with pain and swelling.

Once you know the medical properties of herbs, you can better decide what to use in your liniments. Use a combination of herbs.

Herbal Infused Oils

Herbal oils can be made using various methods, depending on whether you use fresh or dried herbs and what you want to use for the oil. If you plan on making edible essential oil, then you should infuse the oil with fresh herbs. You can infuse any oil, but olive oil and fractionated coconut oil are recommended because they have long shelf lives. To use dried herbs, you must use the alcohol intermediary method. This oil is far more shelf-stable but has an unpleasant taste and is only suitable for external use. If your oil goes rancid, grows mold, or changes over time, discard it.

Fresh Infused Oil

Ingredients:

- Fresh herbs
- Olive oil, or coconut oil

Method:

1. Put the herbs in a clean, dry jar. Leave 1-3 inches of space above the herbs.
2. Fill the jar with oil, covering the herbs with at least 1 inch of oil. Cap the jar and shake vigorously.
3. Put the jar on a warm, sunny windowsill and shake it at least once daily.
4. After 2–3 weeks, strain the herbs using a cheesecloth.
5. Pour into clean glass bottles and label them with the date, oil, and herbs. For up to a year, store in a cool, dark place.

Notes:

You can make herbal oil more quickly by cooking the herbs in the oil at 100°–140°F for 1–5 hours. You have to be careful not to fry the herbs. You can store this oil for up to 6 months.

You can add vitamin E oil at a concentration of up to 1% to extend the shelf life of your oil, but it will not be edible.

Alcohol Intermediary Method

Ingredients:

- 1 ounce of dried herbs
- ½ ounce of grain alcohol or vodka
- 8 ounces of oil

Method:

1. Grind the herbs into a coarse powder and put them in a clean jar. Top with the alcohol and shake or mix to combine. Set aside for 24 hours.
2. Put the soaked herbs into a blender along with the oil. Blend for 5 minutes or until the blender jar is warm.
3. Pour the mixture through a cheesecloth-lined strainer into a bowl. You may need to strain the mixture again through a coffee filter for more precise results.

4. Store the oils in glass bottles in a cool, dark place. Don't forget to label it.

Notes:

This oil isn't edible but will have a longer shelf life.

Salves

Herbal salves are a gentle topical treatment for scrapes and rashes and can moisturize dry skin. A salve is made from herbal oils, such as those mentioned above, in combination with beeswax. It can then be rubbed onto the skin to get the beneficial effects of the herbs and the soothing effects of the wax.

Ingredients:

- 8 ounces of infused herbal oil
- 1-ounce beeswax (grated or pellets)
- Optional: essential oils of your choice

Method:

1. Warm the oil in a double boiler or a heatproof bowl over a saucepan of simmering water, and then add the beeswax. Stir until melted.
2. Test the consistency of the salve by putting a clean spoon in the freezer. Dip it into the salve and see how it sets. If it's softer than you'd like, add more

beeswax.

3. Pour the warm salve into containers. Add any essential oils and stir with a chopstick.

4. For up to a year, store in a cool, dark place.

5. Notes: You can make salves of plantain, yarrow, mint, nettle leaves, creosote bush, chickweed, pine needles, comfrey, dandelion, arnica, echinacea , chamomile, and lavender.

Poultices

In short, a poultice is a way to directly apply herbs to the skin. The herbs are typically mashed with water or oil to produce a paste. It might be rubbed on the skin, placed in a cloth bag, pressed against it, or put on a bandage. Depending on what herbs make up a poultice and whether it's hot or cold, it can increase circulation or relieve pain from a sunburn or insect bite. Herbs can fight infection, reduce inflammation, relieve aching muscles, or soothe congestion. You can use many different herbs to make a poultice, but plantain leaves, chickweed leaves, and dandelion leaves are often used. That's because they're easy to find and harvest, safe, and known for their healing properties.

A simple way to make a poultice is to put the herbs into a muslin bag and tie a knot to close the bag. Then place it in a bowl of hot water and knead it for a minute or so before applying the bag to the affected area. You can also make a poultice by combining the herbs with a bit of water and mashing it into a pulp before rubbing it onto your skin and wrapping it with a bandage or plastic wrap.

Sitz Bath

A sitz bath is a shallow bath with salt, herbs, and other beneficial ingredients that can relieve pain and fatigue. The sitz bath comes from the German "sitzen," which means "to sit." The combination of warm water and the other ingredients provides a relaxing and therapeutic experience, especially if your muscles or joints are sore. You can use dried, powdered, or fresh herbs in your sitz bath. Good options include:

- Chamomile flowers
- Lavender
- Rosemary leaves
- Sage leaves
- Ground ginger
- St. John's wort
- Comfrey leaves

Ingredients:

- 1-2 cups of Epsom salt per gallon of water
- ½-¾ cups of baking soda per gallon of water
- Optional: 1 cup of other salts, such as Himalayan pink rock salt
- ½ cup of herbs in a muslin bag

Method:

1. Clean out your bathtub of any soap residue and add water. It should be warm enough to dissolve the salt without being uncomfortable. Aim for enough water to cover your hips when you sit down.
2. Add the other ingredients and agitate the water to dissolve the salts and baking soda, allowing the herbal qualities to permeate the water.
3. Soak for 15-20 minutes or so.
4. Rinse the salt from your body and the bathtub with clean water.

Now that we've looked at what you can do with the medicinal plants you've harvested, it's time to explore what you can. The following section will discuss 127 herbal plant profiles found in the American Southwest.

PART II

127 MEDICINAL PLANT PROFILES

N ow that you know how to harvest and use plants you can find in the wild, here are profiles of some common and valuable medicinal plants in the Southwestern United States. The plant profiles are arranged alphabetically and provide a quick snapshot of what you're likely to find and where. The end of the this chapter QR code for plants photos on page 196.

1. Agrimony

- Scientific name: *Rosaceae Agrimoni.*
- Other names: Common agrimonia, church steeples, sticklewort
- Description: Yellow, five-petaled flowers grow on tall spikes and develop seed pods.
- Location: temperate grasslands in most states

- Season: summer.
- Medicinal uses: as an astringent and wound healer. relieves pain and tension. It helps the gallbladder, liver, bladder, and kidneys.
- Parts used: flowers and seeds
- Preparations/Dosage: Tea infusion drink three times a day. Tincture take 1-4 ml three times a day.
- **Caution: It may exacerbate constipation.**

2. Alder

- Scientific name: *Alnus incana*
- Other names: Arizona alder
- Description: Deciduous small-medium trees with simple, alternate, serrated leaves and smooth, gray bark. grows catkins in early spring.
- Location: Arizona New Mexico
- Season: spring
- Medicinal uses: Treats stomach aches.
- Parts used: bark.
- Preparations/Dosage: Boil bark in water for tea.

3. American Licorice

- Scientific name: *Glycyrrhiza lepidota*
- Other names: wild licorice.
- Description: It reaches up to 39 inches tall and has simple leaves, white flowers, and tough brown roots.

- Location: Found in Texas and California.
- Season: Fall.
- Medicinal uses: Treats respiratory infections, skin problems, and heartburn, relieving stress, balancing hormones.
- Parts used: roots
- Preparations/Dosage: Boil the root into a tea. Apply licorice extract externally for skin conditions. Take ½ teaspoon of tincture twice a day for respiratory or gastric issues.
- **Caution: It may interact with medications or preexisting conditions. Avoid if pregnant or breastfeeding. Consult a doctor before using it medicinally.**

4. Anemone

- Scientific name: *Anemone tuberosa.*
- Other names: desert anemone.
- Description: Has basal leaves and pinkish-white flowers. grows woody tubers.
- Location: Nevada, New Mexico, Western California, and Texas
- Season: spring or fall.
- Medicinal uses for panic attacks and anxiety
- Parts used: tubers/roots.
- Preparations/Dosage: Create a tincture and use 5–10 drops when needed.

- **Caution: Fumes can be caustic when blending fresh plants.**

5. Antelope Horns

- Scientific name: *Asclepias asperula.*
- Other names: antelope horn milkweed, spider milkweed.
- Description: Clustered, greenish-yellow flowers and seed pods that resemble antelope horns.
- Location: Southwestern US
- Season: fall.
- Medicinal uses: heart health, lung health, high fever, eye problems, headaches.
- Parts used: roots. Seeds and flowers are edible.
- Preparations/Dosage: Dry and powder the root and make it into a tea. Take it daily.
- **Caution: Avoid large quantities. Avoid if pregnant.**

6. Arizona cypress

- Scientific Name: *Cupressus arizonica*
- Description: An evergreen tree with scalelike leaves and globular cones.
- Location: Southwestern US.
- Medicinal uses: include detoxifying lymph systems, relaxing muscles, and treating coughs and colds.
- Parts used: branches, leaves, cones, and oil.

- Preparations/Dosage: Dry leaves for tea otherwise, make extract for foot soaks, salves, and soothing baths.

7. Ash

- Scientific Name: *Fraxinus*
- Description: Medium to large deciduous trees with opposite, pinnately compound leaves and helicopter leaves. Most ash species have pale gray bark.
- Location: Different species grow throughout the US.
- Season: spring.
- Medicinal uses: fever, arthritis, gout, constipation, fluid retention, bladder problems, menstrual cramps, circulation issues.
- Parts used: bark.
- Preparations/Dosage: Boil the roots to make tea.
- **Caution: As usual, speak to a doctor if you have any preexisting conditions.**

8. Aspen

- Scientific name: *Populus tremuloides*
- Other names: American aspen, white poplar, trembling aspen.
- Description: A deciduous tree with white bark and rounded leaves.
- Location: Found throughout the US.

- Season: spring.
- Medicinal uses: can treat wounds, skin conditions, respiratory disorders, or be used as a pain reliever.
- Parts used: bark and leaves.
- Preparations/Dosage: Make tea by boiling the bark in water. You can also create an ointment for topical use.
- **Caution: Avoid if you have an aspirin allergy.**

9. Beardtongue

- Scientific name: *Penstemon*
- Description: Has distinctive tube-shaped, two lipped flowers with a prominent infertile stamen, often giving the appearance of a hairy tongue.
- Location: Different species grow throughout the US.
- Season: fall.
- Medicinal uses: chest pains, stomach aches, fevers.
- Parts used: roots and leaves.
- Preparations/Dosage: Boil the roots or leaves to create tea.

10. Lemon Beebalm

- Scientific name: *Monarda citriodora*
- Other names: lemon bergamot, lemon mint.

- Description: Has lance-shaped leaves that smell of lemons when crushed. has small white, purple, or pink flowers that grow in clusters.
- Location: Southwestern US.
- Season: spring to fall.
- Medicinal uses: Treats coughs, colds, fevers, and other respiratory problems.
- Parts used: leaves
- Preparations/Dosage: Make tea with the leaves. You can also eat it and create an essential oil for insect repellent.

11. Bermudagrass

- Scientific name: *Cynodon dactylon*
- Other names: dog's tooth grass, ethena grass, devil's grass.
- Description: Has gray-green short leaf blades with rough edges. The stems are flat and tinged purple.
- Location: California and other southern US states.
- Season: Fall.
- Medicinal uses: Acts as a diuretic, antibiotic, antiseptic, and aperient.
- Parts used: roots and grass.
- Preparations/Dosage: Make a tea by boiling the roots. You can also juice the grass to create an astringent.

12. Betony

- Scientific name: *Pedicularis canadensis*
- Other names: wood betony, bishopwort.
- Description: This plant has soft, hairy basal leaves that are deeply toothed. produces clusters of hooded flowers on spikes.
- Location: Texas.
- Season: fall.
- Medicinal uses: treats heartburn, gastritis, colds, and sinusitis.
- Parts used: roots.
- Preparations/Dosage: Create a root infusion. You can also make a poultice for sore muscles. It is also edible.

13. Blackberry

- Scientific Name: *Rubus fruticosus*
- Description: has thorny canes. grows white flowers that mature into black aggregate fruits.
- Location: found throughout the US.
- Season: summer and fall.
- Medicinal uses: used to treat cancer, dysentery, diarrhea, whooping cough, colitis, toothache, and anemia. has antioxidant and anti-inflammatory properties.

- Parts Used: Fruits are eaten, and leaves and roots are used medicinally.
- Preparations/Dosage: Make tea with the leaves and roots. You can also create an herbal extract or blackberry capsules.
- **Caution: Pregnant or breastfeeding women and children under two years of age should avoid tea.**

14. Blazing Star

- Scientific Name: *Liatris aestivalis*
- Other names: summer blazing star, summer gayfeather.
- Description: leathery leaves and purple flowers grow in clusters on spikes. The roots are tuberous.
- Location: found in Texas and Oklahoma.
- Season: fall.
- Medicinal uses: treats pain, headaches, arthritis, earaches, fever, and upset stomach.
- Parts used: roots and leaves.
- Preparations/Dosage: the roots can be boiled into tea or dried and ground into a powder for capsules. The leaves can also be made into tea for an upset stomach.

15. Brickellbush

- Scientific name: *Brickellia*

- Other names: Terlingua bricklebush
- Description: woody, perennial shrubs with small leaves and clusters of narrow, cylindrical flower heads.
- Location: Southwestern US
- Medicinal uses: treats fever, skin issues, respiratory issues, and stomach problems; can be used for type 2 (non-insulin-dependent diabetes).
- Parts used: leaves and stems.
- Preparations/Dosage: Steep to make tea.
- **Caution: Unsuitable for anyone with type-1 diabetes.**

16. Brittlebush

- Scientific name: *Encelia farinosa*
- Other names: incienso, a desert shrub.
- Description: drought deciduous with thick, brittle stems. had small, fragrant leaves and yellow or purple flowers.
- Location: Southwestern US
- Medicinal uses: Toothache, chest pain
- Parts used: Stems
- Preparations/Dosage: remove the bark, heat the stem, and place it on the tooth. Heat the gum in the stem and apply it to the chest for chest pain.

17. Buttonbush

- Scientific name: *Cephalanthus occidentalis*
- Other names: button willow, buck brush, honey bells.
- Description: deciduous shrub with dense, spherical white or pale yellow flowers.
- Location: Arizona.
- Medicinal uses: Bark is an astringent used to treat stomach issues. Roots and fruit can treat constipation. Leaves are astringent and diuretic.
- Parts used: bark, roots, fruits, and leaves.
- Preparations/Dosage: boil the bark, roots, or fruit into a tea. steep the leaves
- **Caution: Leaves are toxic in large quantities.**

18. California Poppy

- Scientific name: *Eschscholzia california*
- Other names: golden poppies, a cup of gold, California sunlight.
- Description: It reaches about 2 feet tall and has bright flowers with four petals that range from yellow to pink, orange, or red.
- Location: California, Nevada, Arizona, New Mexico
- Season: summer.
- Medicinal uses: Treats anxiety, used as a painkiller and mild sedative.

- Parts used: flowers and leaves.
- Preparations/Dosage: Create an infused tea with the leaves and flowers. You can also make a liquid extract or capsules.
- **Caution: Take in moderation.**

19. Camphorweed

- Scientific name: *Heterotheca subaxillaris*
- Other names: Mexican arnica.
- Description: a herb with tall, erect, hairy stems. has yellow flowers.
- Location: found throughout the US.
- Medicinal uses: relieves gas, diarrhea, and menstrual cramps. It can be used as an antifungal and antiseptic wash.
- Parts used: the whole plant
- Preparations/Dosage: Create an herb oil to use topically. Dry the plant to use in teas.

20. Canyon Bursage

- Scientific name: *Ambrosia ambrosioides*
- Other names: Canyon ragweed.
- Description: Shrug with coarsely-toothed leaves, multiple erect hairy stems, and yellowish-green flowers.
- Location: Arizona.

- Medicinal uses: analgesic; treats menstrual cramps. Leaf poultice loosens the cough.
- Parts used: roots and leaves.
- Preparations/Dosage: Crush the roots and boil them in water for a soothing tea. Warm and crush the leaves for a poultice.

21. Cattail

- Scientific name: *Typha.*
- Other names: reeds, punks.
- Description:Semi-aquatic, with a tall, erect stem and a flowering spike. The flowers grow as a tight, sausage-shaped brown cluster that matures into cotton-like fluff.
- Location: wetlands throughout North America.
- Season: fall.
- Medicinal uses: edible diuretic. used externally to treat sores, boils, wounds, burns, and scabs.
- Parts used: roots and flowers
- Preparations/Dosage: boil the rootstock to use as a diuretic. Mash into a paste to use topically.

22. Cascara Sagrada

- Scientific name: *Rhamnus purshiana.*
- Other names: Cascara buckthorn, bearberry, holy bark, bearwood.

- Description: dark, smooth, reddish bark with oblong leaves and red or black berries (depending on the season).
- Location: Northwestern US
- Season: fall.
- Medicinal uses: laxative
- Parts used: bark
- Preparations/Dosage: Steep for an infusion, or take as small a dose of liquid extract as possible.
- **Caution: Use for no longer than a week. Long-term use can cause liver damage. Pregnant women, breastfeeding women, and anyone on other medications shouldn't use them.**

23. Chaste tree

- Scientific Name: *Vitex agnus castus*
- Other names: chasteberry, vitex
- Description: Prefers brackish water. small tree with aromatic leaves and spikes of lavender flowers in summer
- Location: Texas
- Season: summer and fall
- Medicinal uses: reproductive health issues
- Parts used: leaves, flowers, and berries
- Preparations/Dosage: Take as a decoction, tincture, or vinegar tincture.

- **Caution: This can cause adverse effects or interfere with medications. Do not take it while pregnant or breastfeeding.**

24. Chia

- Scientific name: *Salvia hispanica*
- Description: An annual herb with opposite leaves and purple or white flowers that grow in clusters on spikes. The seeds are oval and 1 mm in diameter.
- Location: Southwestern US.
- Season: summer and fall.
- Medicinal uses: protects against cardiovascular disease and diabetes.
- Parts used: Seeds
- Preparations/Dosage: Grind the seeds to use as a food supplement. Take no more than 48 g per day.

25. Chickweed

- Scientific name: *Stellaria media*
- Other names: chickenwort, craches, maruns, winter weed
- Description: Large mats of ground foliage with slender stems and a distinctive hair line. small oval leaves and tiny white flowers.
- Location: Throughout the US
- Season: winter and early spring.

- Medicinal uses: Treats skin conditions, pulmonary diseases, bruises, and pain.
- Parts used: stems and leaves
- Preparations/Dosage: steep in hot water, then apply externally, make salves.

26. Chicory

- Scientific name: *Cichorium intybus*
- Other names: blue daisy, blue dandelion
- Description: An herb with hairy stems and distinctive bright purplish-blue flowers.
- Location: throughout the US.
- Season: fall.
- Medicinal uses: include treating liver problems, heart disease, constipation, swelling, and sinus infections.
- Parts used: leaves and roots.
- Preparations/Dosage: Eat the leaves raw. Boil the tea for an infusion. Crushed leaves may treat fungal skin conditions. You can also make a tincture or create capsules from dried roots.
- **Caution: It may cause skin irritation. Avoid it during pregnancy, while breastfeeding, or if you have gallstones.**

27. Chokecherry

- Scientific name: *Prunus virginiana*
- Other names: bitterberry, Virginia bird cherry.
- Description: shrug with oval, serrated leaves and small white flowers that grow in clusters. Fruits are dark red or black and astringent.
- Location: throughout the US, New Mexico.
- Season: fall.
- Medicinal uses: astringent, sedative, appetite stimulant, treats fevers, coughs, stomach aches, and colds. It can be used externally as a wash for burns, sores, and ulcers.
- Parts used: inner bark and roots.
- Preparations/Dosage: Create a tea from the bark. Make an infusion of root bark for a topical wash.
- **Caution: Fruit stones and leaves are poisonous.**

28. Cholla

- Scientific name: *Cylindropuntia*
- Description: Cacti with thin, cylindrical, branching stem segments instead of pads. It usually has dense spines and bristles.
- Location: Southwestern US.
- Medicinal uses: burns, gastrointestinal disorders, urinary tract problems.
- Parts used: fleshy stem and sap.

- Preparations/Dosage: Fruits and buds are edible. Roast the stem flesh and apply it to burns as a topical poultice.
- **Caution: Beware of the spines.**

29. Cleavers

- Scientific name: *Galium aparine*
- Other names: sticky weed, catchweed, sticky jack
- Description:A creeping plant with tiny hooked hairs on the stems and leaves that stick to animal fur and clothing.
- Location: found throughout the US.
- Season: spring and summer
- Medicinal uses: treats skin conditions, wounds, and burns.
- Parts used: entire plant
- Preparations/Dosage: The leaves can be dried and made into tea. The whole plant can be mashed and used as a poultice.
- **Caution: It can cause dermatitis in some people.**

30. Cocklebur

- Scientific name: *Xanthium strumarium*
- Other names: rough cocklebur, common cocklebur
- Description: shrub with distinctive spiny, cylindrical green burs that grow directly from the stem.

- Location: Southwestern desert areas.
- Medicinal uses: used to treat rhinitis, nasal sinusitis, headaches, ulcers, and arthritis. The root can treat fever.
- Parts used: fruits and roots.
- Preparations/Dosage: bake the fruits to a yellowish color. Boil the root into a tea.
- **Caution: Only use small amounts; large quantities are toxic.**

31. Copperleaf

- Scientific name: *Acalypha neomexicana.*
- Other names: three-seeded mercury, New Mexico copperleaf.
- Description: An herb with erect, golden-red stems. greenish leaves and green flowers that grow on spikes.
- Location: New Mexico
- Medicinal uses: Heals wounds and ulcers.
- Parts used: leaves and stems.
- Preparations/Dosage: Create a poultice and use it topically.

32. Cottonwood

- Scientific name: *Populus sect. Aigeiros.*

- Description: Large deciduous trees with thick, fissured bark and diamond-shaped leaves. grows catkins in the spring before leaves arrive.
- Location: Texas, Arizona, Nevada, New Mexico, Utah
- Season: Spring.
- Medicinal uses: reduces fever, inflammation, and pain.
- Parts used: flower buds.
- Preparations/Dosage: Make cottonwood bud oil for topical uses. Add to baths or apply directly to the skin.
- **Caution: Avoid being allergic to bees or aspirin.**

33. Cow parsnip

- Scientific name: *Heracleum maximum.*
- Other names: Indian celery, Indian rhubarb, pushki.
- Description: tall herbaceous plants with hollow, hairy stems and distinctive white flower umbels that grow in clusters. See diagram 3 (page 65)
- Location: California, New Mexico.
- Medicinal uses: Treats bruises or sores.
- Parts used: roots and leaves.
- Preparations/Dosage: Heat the leaves and root and add to healing poultices.

- **Caution: Young leaves are toxic, and the sap may cause scarring rashes when exposed to UV light. Do not mistake it for giant hogweed or hemlock.**

34. Cranesbill

- Scientific name: *Geranium.*
- Description: Flowering plant with cleft leaves and five-petaled white, pink, blue, or purple flowers.
- Location: Different species are found throughout the US.
- Season: spring and summer.
- Medicinal uses: Treats ulcers and acts as an expectorant. Repels insects.
- Parts used: leaves.
- Preparations/Dosage: Make an herbal oil out of leaves. Make tea with the leaves or create a compress.
- **Caution: It may cause contact dermatitis.**

35. Creosote Bush

- Scientific name: *Larrea tridentata*
- Other names: greasewood, jarillas, chaparral
- Description: A flowering shrub with dark green leaves and round, yellow flowers.
- Location: Southwestern US.
- Medicinal uses: treats wounds, sores, stiff limbs, and cramps. It is an emetic.

- Parts used: leaves.
- Preparations/Dosage: Boil the leaves to use as a poultice. The tea is an emetic.
- **Caution: Extensive internal use may damage the liver and kidneys.**

36. Cudweed

- Scientific name: *Diaperia verna.*
- Other names: spring pygmy cudweed, spring rabbit tobacco.
- Description: Herb with greenish-gray hairy leaves and white flowers.
- Location: Arizona, New Mexico, Oklahoma, Texas.
- Medicinal uses: Treats high blood pressure, stomach ulcers, diarrhea, and gastrointestinal distress.
- Parts used: Flowers, leaves, stems.
- Preparations/Dosage: Steep to make tea.

37. Curly Dock

- Scientific name: *Rumex crispus*
- Other names: yellow dock, curled dock.
- Description: Herbaceous with a taproot and a tall, slender, erect stem. Has distinctive pointed green leaves with curled edges.
- Location: Throughout the US.
- Season: summer and fall.

- Medicinal uses: Laxative, reduces inflammation, and treats vascular disorders.
- Parts used: roots, leaves.
- Preparations/Dosage: Dry the roots and boil them as tea. The leaves can be boiled into tea as well or cooked and eaten. A root decoction can also be applied topically.
- **Caution: Extensive use as a laxative causes dependency. Consuming large amounts of uncooked leaves can be toxic.**

38. Dandelion

- Scientific name: *Taraxacium officinale*
- Other names: common dandelion
- Description: A common plant with a thick stem and milky sap. The basal leaves are deeply toothed, and the yellow flowers mature into fluffy white seed clusters. See diagram 1 (page 63)
- Location: Throughout the US.
- Season: Spring.
- Medicinal uses: diuretics promote liver and gastrointestinal health.
- Parts used: flower, leaves and roots.
- Preparations/Dosage: The leaves can be cooked or eaten raw. The roots can be boiled into a decoction or roasted and steeped as tea or a substitute for coffee. The whole plant can be turned into a

tincture, Flower head steep to tea, infused oil and salve.

- **Caution: Some medications may be affected.**

39. Desert Cotton

- Scientific name: *Gossypium thurberi*
- Other names: Arizona wild cotton, Thurber's cotton.
- Description: Perennial shrub with palmately green leaves and pale yellow petalled flowers.
- Location: Arizona and New Mexico.
- Season: summer and fall.
- Medicinal uses: Anti-inflammation, especially in the female reproductive system, supports hormone balance
- Parts used: root bark, and seeds.
- Preparations/Dosage: The root and bark can be boiled into a decoction and made into a tincture. You can grind seed to meal and use it as a food supplement.
- **Caution: Do not be used by pregnant women.**

40. Desert Lavender

- Scientific name: *Condea emoryi*
- Description: Shrub with hairy, pale gray-green oval leaves and small, aromatic lavender flowers.
- Location: Southwestern desert areas.

- Medicinal uses: Treats acid reflux, gastric ulcers, and liver complaints, including hangovers. Soothes anxiety.
- Parts used: leaves and flowers.
- Preparations/Dosage: Turn into a tea for quick treatments or create a tincture, and salve.
- **Caution: Do not overharvest; this is a slow-growing herb.**

41. Desert Willow

- Scientific name: *Chilopsis linearis*
- Other names: catalpa willow,desert catalpa ,false willow, flowering willow
- Description: shrub or small tree with willow-like, narrow deciduous leaves. blooms purple-pink flowers in the summer
- Location: Southwestern US
- Medicinal uses: Treats fungal infections and promotes cardiovascular health. also used for wounds and coughs.
- Parts used: flowers, leaves, and bark.
- Preparations/Dosage: The flowers, leaves, and bark can be made into a poultice for topical use. The flowers can be made into an antioxidant-rich tea.

42. Dewberry (Southern)

- Scientific name: *Rubus trivialis*
- Other names: Dewberry
- Description: It looks similar to blackberries, but the stems trail along the ground instead of forming upright canes.
- Location: Texas, Oklahoma, Look for open woodlands, meadows, and disturbed areas.
- Season: fall
- Medicinal uses: Roots treat diarrhea and rheumatism, used externally for piles. Leaves regulate urination.
- Parts used: roots, leaves, and fruits
- Preparations/Dosage: Boil the roots to use internally and externally. A decoction of the leaves makes tea.

43. Echinacea

- Scientific name: *Echinacea purpurea*
- Other names: purple coneflower.
- Description: An herb that grows individual stems with hairy leaves that terminate in a purplish-pink flower
- Location: Texas and throughout the US
- Season: summer and fall

- Medicinal uses: treats colds, sore throats, muscle pain, respiratory and urinary tract infections, and strengthens immunity
- Parts used: the whole plant
- Preparations/Dosage: Can be consumed raw or brewed into a tea. You can process it into an essential oil, a tincture, or capsules.

44. Elder

- Scientific name: *Sambucus nigra*
- Other names: elderberry, black elder
- Description: Shrub with gray bark and large clusters of flowers that ripen into dropping clusters of black berries in fall.
- Location: Throughout the US.
- Season: summer and fall.
- Medicinal uses: treats cold and flu symptoms.
- Parts used: flowers and fruits.
- Preparations/Dosage: Create a herbal extract or tincture.
- **Caution: Raw berries and foliage are toxic.**

45. Estafiate

- Scientific name: *Artemisia ludoviciana*
- Other names: Western mugwort, mountain sage, white sage, prairie sage

- Description: Stems and long leaves are covered in gray or white hair. On top of the stem grows a narrow cluster of hanging flower heads.
- Location: throughout US
- Medicinal uses: Treats skin conditions, colds, fevers, and sore throats.
- Parts used: leaves
- Preparations/Dosage: dry the leaves and use them for medicinal tea. You can also use it as an herb.

46. Evening Primrose

- Scientific name: *Oenothera biennis*
- Other names: common evening primrose.
- Description: biennial plant with spiraling leaves and yellow flowers that grow on a tall spike.
- Location: Texas
- Medicinal uses: treats eczema, arthritis, menstrual cramps, and menopausal symptoms, among other conditions.
- Parts used: the whole plant
- Preparations/Dosage: used to make a herbal oil, tincture, or tea to be ingested. The roots can be used topically to treat boils.
- **Caution: May worsen bleeding disorders.**

47. Fanpetals

- Scientific name: *Sida*
- Other names: spreading panpetals
- Description: shrubs with hairy stems and leaves. They have serrated leaves and small yellow flowers.
- Location: Southwestern US
- Season: fall.
- Medicinal uses: antiseptic and anti-inflammatory, treats fever, wounds, infections, stomach, and respiratory issues.
- Parts used: leaves and roots
- Preparations/Dosage: Leaves can be cooked and eaten. Both leaves and roots can be boiled for tea.

48. Feverfew

- Scientific name: *Tanacetum parthenium*
- Description: A small bush with daisy-like flowers and pungent leaves.
- Location: Throughout the US.
- Medicinal uses: Treats headache, pain, and fever.
- Parts used: leaves.
- Preparations/Dosage: Steep the fresh or dried leaves for tea. Concentrated tinctures at 1 ml a day (up to 60 drops) can lower fevers. Topical salves can help the skin. Feverfew oil can help stiff muscles.

- **Caution: Long-term use may lead to dependence. Can interact with medications.**

49. Figwort

- Scientific name: *Scrophularia desertorum*
- Other names: Desert figwort.
- Description: Perennial herb with clusters of erect stems and long leaf stems. The hooded flowers grow in clusters on hairy branches.
- Location: California and Nevada.
- Medicinal uses; skin conditions like eczema, itching, piles, and acne.
- Parts used: the whole plant.
- Preparations/Dosage: Create an infusion to drink up to 3 times a day or a tincture. You can also apply it topically as part of a salve or poultice.

50. Filaree

- Scientific name: *Erodium cicutarium.*
- Other names: stork's bill, redstem filaree, pinweed.
- Description: This is a hairy, sticky plant with reddish stems and bright pink flowers.
- Location: Southwestern US, in desert and arid areas.
- Season: fall.
- Medicinal uses: sores, rashes, and stomach aches.
- Parts used: roots

- Preparations/Dosage: Create a topical poultice for sores and rashes. A root infusion is used internally for stomach aches.

51. Fireweed

- Scientific name: *Chamaenerion angustifolium*
- Other names: willowherb, rosebay willowherb.
- Description: Tall, erect stems with simple, scattered leaves terminate in a cluster of small purple flowers.
- Location: throughout the US
- Medicinal uses: treats migraines, colds, stomach ulcers, inflammation, and promotes wound healing.
- Parts used: aerial parts.
- Preparations/Dosage: leaves are fermented, dried, and brewed into tea.

52. Globemallow

- Scientific name: *Sphaeralcea ambigua.*
- Other names: Desert globemallow, apricot mallow.
- Description: a small shrub with fuzzy, white-haired leaves. Grows bowl-shaped orange flowers in spring that mature into brown spherical fruits.
- Location: Arizona, California, Nevada, Utah
- Season: spring and fall.
- Medicinal uses: Treats colds, coughs, and diarrhea. used topically for snake bites, wounds, and arthritis.

It can reduce inflammation and boost the immune system.
- Parts used: roots, leaves, flowers.
- Preparations/Dosage: The roots can be made into a poultice to be used topically. The leaves and flowers can be dried and steeped for tea.
- **Caution: Strain the tea, the leaf hairs may irritate the throat.**

53. Goatbush

- Scientific name: *Castela erecta subsp. texana.*
- Other names: allthorn, allthorn castela, bisbirinda, Texas goatbush
- Description: A medium shrub with thorn-tipped branch, and bitter, silvery leaves, and tiny red flowers that mature into flattened, bright red fruits.
- Location: Texas.
- Season: fall.
- Medicinal uses: Treats intestinal problems, fever, colic, and parasites.
- Parts used: leaves and bark.
- Preparations/Dosage: You can make a bitter tea with the leaves or create an extract from the bark.
- **Caution: Beware of thorns when harvesting.**

54. Goldenrod

- Scientific name: *Solidago odora.*
- Other names: blue mountain tea
- Description: A fairly smooth-stemmed herb with narrow, pointed, fragrant leaves and small yellow flowers in summer and fall.
- Location: Southwestern US and Texas
- Season: summer and fall.
- Medicinal uses: treats digestive problems, sore throats, and coughs.
- Parts used: leaves and flowers.
- Preparations/Dosage: steep or infuse for tea, make tincture.

55. Golden Smoke

- Scientific name: *Cotinus coggygria*
- Other names: smoke bush, smoke tea.
- Description: deciduous shrub with multiple branches and waxy green leaves. Flowers grow in large clusters and can form yellow or pink feathery plumes.
- Location: Oklahoma, Texas.
- Medicinal uses: can treat eye issues, digestive problems, and fever.
- Parts used: leaves and flowers.
- Preparations/Dosage: Create an essential oil.

- **Caution: It may cause dermatitis if sensitive.**

56. Gumweed

- Scientific name: *Grindelia squarrosa*
- Other names: curly-top gumweed.
- Description: An erect, branching herb with gray-green resinous leaves. produces yellow ray flowers.
- Location: Western, Central, and parts of the Southern US.
- Season: summer and fall.
- Medicinal uses: Treats lung complaints and skin rashes.
- Parts used: flowers, leaves, resin.
- Preparations/Dosage: Resin is used topically for poison ivy rashes. Flowers and leaves can be used to make a tincture.
- **Caution: Can be toxic when ingested.**

57. Hackberry

- Scientific Name: *Celtis occidentalis.*
- Other names: nettle tree, sugarberry, beaver wood.
- Description: Medium-sized tree with cork-like, warty bark. Green, pointed leaves produce small orange or purple fruits in the fall.
- Location: Oklahoma, Texas
- Season: fall.

- Medicinal uses: regulates menstrual cycles and treats sore throats.
- Parts used: bark; fruit is edible.
- Preparations/Dosage: Create a decoction of the bark.

58. Hawthorn

- Scientific name: *Crataegus.*
- Other names: quickthorn, thornapple, may-tree, hawberry.
- Description: Shrubs or small trees with thorny branches. It has gray bark that may be smooth or narrowly ridged. produces white flowers that mature into berry-like fruits.
- Location: Throughout the US.
- Medicinal uses: digestive aid and strengthen the heart.
- Parts used: leaves, flowers, and fruit.
- Preparations/Dosage: Eat fresh or dried fruits. Can be made as a tea with leaves and flowers.
- **Caution: Overdosing can cause low blood pressure. avoid it if you take digoxin.**

59. Hopbush

- Scientific name: *Dodonaea viscosa.*
- Other names: Hopseed bush.

- Description: Shrub with broad, resinous, leathery leaves. produces yellow, orange, or red flowers and produces brown-winged fruit.
- Location: Arizona, Nevada, California.
- Medicinal uses: it heals wounds, rashes, and insect bites. Also treats sore throats and fevers.
- Parts used: stems, and leaves.
- Preparations/Dosage: Create a poultice for topical applications or make a tea infusion.

60. Hoptree

- Scientific name: *Ptelea trifoliata*
- Other names: Wafer ash, skunk bush.
- Description: Deciduous shrub with a few spreading stems. Has reddish or gray-brown bark and an unpleasant smell.
- Location: Nevada, Arizona.
- Season: fall.
- Medicinal uses: Promotes appetite, treats fevers, digestive issues, parasites, and wounds.
- Parts used: Roots and leaves
- Preparations/Dosage: Create a tonic or decoction for internal use. The leaves can be made into a poultice.

61. Horsetail

- Scientific name: *Equisetum arvense*

- Other names: horse willow, snake grass, shave grass, toadpipe, scouring rush, bottlebrush.
- Description: Resembles a horse's tail, with clusters of branching upright stems. Anceint tree like plants
- Location: Throughout the US.
- Medicinal uses: Diuretic, promotes kidney health, heals wounds, bone fractures and osteoporosis.
- Parts used: Stem.
- Preparations/Dosage: Dry and create an infusion for tea 2-3 tsp 3 times daily or make a tincture (1:5). Apply decoction or tincture externally to small wounds and scratches.
- **Caution: Don't use it for an extended time. Contains nicotine. Interacts with alcohol and other drugs/medication.**

62. Horseweed

- Scientific name: *Erigeron canadensis*
- Other names: Canadian horseweed, fleabane, butterweed.
- Description: Has sparsely hairy stems and unstalked, toothed leaves that spiral up the erect stem. Flowers grow in clusters.
- Location: Throughout the US.
- Medicinal uses: Sore throat and dysentery can induce sneezing.
- Parts used: Flowers and leaves.

- Preparations/Dosage: Make a tincture or essential oil with the dried flowers. The leaves can be made into tea.

63. Hounds-tongue

- Scientific name: *Cynoglossum officinale*
- Other names: hound's tooth, gypsy flower, dog's tongue.
- Description: An invasive plant with grayish, softly-haired leaves and reddish-purple funnel-shaped flowers.
- Location: Southwestern US.
- Medicinal uses: Treats diarrhea, skin problems, coughs, and wounds.
- Parts used: Leaves.
- Preparations/Dosage: Leaves are mashed and boiled in water to make tea.
- **Caution: Possible carcinogen, toxic to cows.**

64. Immortalle

- Scientific name: *Helichrysum italicum.*
- Other names: Italian strawflower, curry plant.
- Description: Woody stems with clusters of yellow flowers and a curry-like smell of leaves.
- Location: Dry, rocky ground in warm areas. native to the Mediterranean but introduced to the US.

- Medicinal uses: Heals wounds, skin inflammation, and digestive problems. has anti-inflammatory, antibacterial, and antifungal properties.
- Parts used: Leaves, stems, and flowers.
- Preparations/Dosage: Make an herbal oil or steep it in tea.

65. Jojoba

- Scientific name: *Simmondsia chinensis*
- Other names: coffeeberry, goat nut, wild hazel.
- Description: Evergreen shrug with coarse, leathery leaves and small, greenish-yellow flowers.
- Location: Southern California, Arizona.
- Season: summer and fall.
- Medicinal uses: Improves skin, scalp, and hair health.
- Parts used: Seeds.
- Preparations/Dosage: Create a salve for topical applications.
- **Caution: Do not ingest.**

66. Juniper

- Scientific name: *Juniperus*
- Description: Coniferous tree with needle-like leaves and small bluish-purple berries.
- Location: Throughout North America

- Medicinal uses: diuretics, which treat urinary tract infections and help digestion.
- Parts Used: berries
- Preparations/Dosage: Steep the berries for tea or create a tincture. The leaves and berries can be used to make herbal oil.
- **Caution: It interferes with some drugs; excessive doses may cause severe side effects.**

67. Kidneywood

- Scientific name: *Eysenhardtia texana*
- Other names: bee brush, Texas kidneywood.
- Description: Small flowering tree that has small, aromatic flowers and leaves. The small white flowers grow on spikes.
- Location: Texas.
- Medicinal uses: Treats kidney and bladder problems.
- Parts used: Branches.
- Preparations/Dosage: Boil to make tea.

68. Lobelia

- Scientific name: *Lobelia anatina*.
- Other names: apache lobelia, southwestern lobelia
- Description: Small herb with distinctive blueish purple flowers.
- Location: Southwestern US.

- Medicinal uses: Purgative. Treats food poisoning, asthma, and respiratory and muscle disorders. Relaxant.
- Parts used: Leaves.
- Preparations/Dosage: Infuse for tea. Create a tincture to induce vomiting. It can be used topically for muscle spasms.
- **Caution: Excessive use causes vomiting. Use under medical supervision. Avoid it if you have a preexisting condition, pregnant, or are breastfeeding.**

69. Mallow

- Scientific name: *Malva sylvestris*
- Other names: common mallow.
- Description: a herb with heavily lobed and serrated leaves. Has distinctive flowers with five heart-shaped pinkish purple petals and a prominent stamen.
- Location: Throughout the US.
- Medicinal Uses: Reduces pain and swelling and speeds wound healing. Has laxative and diuretic effects.
- Parts Used: Leaves.
- Preparations/Dosage: Make into a hot infusion for tea or create a tincture. A poultice can be applied to wounds.

70. Manzanita

- Scientific name: *Arctostaphylos*
- Description: Evergreen shrubs with orange or red bark and stiff, twisting branches. has small green leaves and edible berries and flowers.
- Location: Western US.
- Medicinal uses: Treats poison oak rashes, urinary tract infections, stomach problems, bronchitis, kidney problems, sores, and headaches.
- Parts used: leaves and berries.
- Preparations/Dosage: make herbal tea for most applications. You can also chew the leaves without swallowing them.

71. Mexican Barberry

- Scientific name: *Berberis haematocarpa*
- Other names: red barberry, Colorado barberry.
- Description: A shrub that has rigid, spiky-toothed leaves that are gray in color and waxy. Produces yellow flowers that mature into edible purplish-red berries.
- Location: Southwestern US
- Season: fall.
- Medicinal uses: Eyewash helps digestive problems and skin conditions (like psoriasis) and acts as a laxative.

- Parts used: roots and fruit.
- Preparations/Dosage: Fruit can be eaten. Wood shavings can be soaked in water for eyewash. The roots can be made into a decoction or a salve. Wood shavings can be soaked in water for eyewash.
- **Caution: Excessive use can cause side effects. Licorice nullifies the effects.**

72. Mexican Palo Verde

- Scientific name: *Parkinsonia aculeata*
- Other names: Jerusalem thorn, jelly bean tree
- Description: Spiny shrub with hairless leaves and stems. Flowers are fragrant and yellow or orange.
- Location: Southwestern US
- Medicinal uses: Treats fever and epilepsy
- Parts used: leaves
- Preparations/Dosage: Steep leaves to make tea.

73. Mimosa

- Scientific name: *Mimosa pudica.*
- Other names: sensitive plant, sleepy plant, action plant, touch-me-not, shame plant.
- Description: Has compound leaves that fold and droop when touched. Produces stalked pinkish-purple ovoid flower heads.
- Location: Texas.

- Medicinal uses: antidepressant, aphrodisiac, diuretic.
- Parts used: the whole plant.
- Preparations/Dosage: Make a tea or tincture.

74. Mock Vervain

- Scientific name: *Glandularia.*
- Other names: mock verbena.
- Description: Has tall stems and showy five-petalled flowers that are either pink, purple, or blue.
- Location: throughout the US.
- Medicinal uses: anti-inflammatory, treats pain, arthritis, gout, colds, skin conditions, and bruising.
- Parts used: aerial parts.
- Preparations/Dosage: Steep in boiling water to make tea. You can also make a poultice or a gargle to soothe a sore throat.

75. Monkey Flower

- Scientific name: *Erythranthe.*
- Other names: musk flowers
- Description: Some plants have a musky odor. Generally, it has glandular leaves and stems and long, tubular flowers. The oval leaves are toothed or lobed.
- Location: western US
- Medicinal uses: as astringents can soothe sore muscles and wounds.

- Parts used: eaves and stems.
- Preparations/Dosage: Create a poultice for topical use or add a decoction to a herbal bath.

76. Mormon Tea

- Scientific name: *Ephedra nevadensis*
- Description: It usually grows as a shrub with green stems and scalelike leaves. Creates pollen cones along the stems.
- Location: Southwestern US states.
- Medicinal uses: treats STDs, colds, and kidney disorders. It's an astringent.
- Parts used: stem.
- Preparations/Dosage: Dry the branches and boil them to make tea.
- **Caution: Other ephedra species contain stimulants linked to severe side effects.**

77. Mulberry

- Scientific name: *Morus.*
- Description: Trees have simple, alternate leaves that are usually lobed or serrated. produces catkins and clustered red or black fruits that hang down.
- Location: throughout the US.
- Season: summer and fall.

- Medicinal uses: beneficial for heart disease, diabetes, and cancer.
- Parts used: fruits.
- Preparations/Dosage: Create an extract, eat raw, or dehydrate and use for tea.
- **Caution: Other plant parts contain toxic milky sap.**

78. Mullein

- Scientific name: *Verbascum thapsus.*
- Other names: velvet plant.
- Description: A herbaceous biennial plant that reaches about 4-6 feet tall. It appears as a rosette of downy, gray leaves in the first year and sprouts clusters of fragrant yellow flowers on a spike in the second year.
- Location: throughout the US.
- Season: summer.
- Medicinal uses: Anti-inflammatory, anti-spasmodic, antimicrobial, soothes pain and treats respiratory infections, warts, and wounds.
- Parts used: flowers.
- Preparations/Dosage: Create a mullein tea for congestion or a poultice for topical use on wounds. You can also create a tincture or essential oil.
- **Caution: Can interfere with anticoagulants.**

79. Nettle

- Scientific name: *Urtica dioica.*
- Other names: common nettle, stinging nettle.
- Description: Hairy stems and soft, toothed leaves that often sting.
- Location: throughout the US.
- Medicinal uses: anti-inflammatory, antihistaminic,
- Parts used: leaves, roots.
- Preparations/Dosage: Cook the leaves and eat. Fresh or dried leaves and roots can be made into tea. You can also make a tincture.
- **Caution: Excessive doses cause side effects. Interacts with some medications and preexisting conditions.**

80. Oat

- Scientific name: *Avena sativa*
- Other names: oatmeal
- Description: Cereal that grows as tall grass. Like other cereals, it produces oat seeds in the summer or fall. See diagram 6 (page 68)
- Location: Throughout the US.
- Season: summer
- Medicinal uses: it lowers blood cholesterol, alleviates constipation, controls blood sugar, treats skin conditions, and has mild antidepressant properties.

- Parts used: oat seeds (harvest when green)
- Preparations/Dosage: Turn into a poultice for skin conditions. You can create a liquid extract from green oats.

81. Ocotillo

- Scientific name: *Fouquieria splendens.*
- Other names: coachwhip, candlewood, Jacob's staff.
- Description: Semi-succulent desert plants that become lush after rainfall with small, ovate leaves and crimson flowers. appears barren otherwise.
- Location: Southwestern US, deserts.
- Season: spring to fall.
- Medicinal uses: relieves fatigue, slows bleeding, alleviates coughing, fluid congestion, UTIs, and varicose veins.
- Parts used: flowers, roots, and bark.
- Preparations/Dosage: Create a tea with the flowers. Soak in bathwater. Create a poultice from flowers and roots. Create a tincture with the bark.

82. Oreganillo

- Scientific name: *Aloysia wrightii.*
- Other names: Wright's beebrush.
- Description: thickly branching rounded shrub with rounded, lightly toothed leaves that have hairy

undersides. Produces a narrow, wooly spike of small white flowers.

- Location: Southwestern US.
- Medicinal uses: stimulates digestion.
- Parts used: flowers and leaves.
- Preparations/Dosage: Create a tea or tincture and take it before meals.

83. Osha

- Scientific name: *Ligusticum porteri.*
- Other names: wild parsnip, porter's lovage, wild celery, Chuchupate and mountain lovage, Colorado cough root,
- Description: Parsley-like leaves and double umbels of white flowers. Leaf bases are reddish. has fibrous roots with dark brown, wrinkly skin and yellowish-white flesh. distinctive spicy celery odor.
- Location: Southwestern US, in the mountains.
- Season: Fall.
- Medicinal uses: Treats colds, sore throats, body aches, fevers, stomach pains, and rheumatism.
- Parts used: root.
- Preparations/Dosage: Use an infusion for body aches. Make tea for internal use.
- **Caution: It has highly toxic lookalikes. The fresh root is highly astringent, potentially blistering the mouth.**

- It's a slow growing plant, so be aware of overharvesting.

84. Oxeye daisy

- Scientific name: *Leucanthemum vulgare.*
- Other names: dog daisy.
- Description: Lower stems have hairy, large leaves at the base that decrease in size further up the stem. blooms up to 3 daisy-like flowers per plant.
- Location: Throughout the US.
- Season: spring, and summer.
- Medicinal uses: Treats lung problems and nervous excitability. Soothes bruises and chapped hands.
- Parts used: flowers.
- Preparations/Dosage: Dry flowers and steep for tea. Create a decoction for an external.

85. Passion flower

- Scientific name: *Passiflora Arizonica, Mexicana*
- Other names: Arizona passion flower, Mexican passion flower
- Description: Long and trailing stems with many tendrils. The lobed leaves are deep green. The distinctive 5-petal flowers are white and purple with five prominent stamens.
- Location: native in Arizona,

- Season: Summer.
- Medicinal uses: sedative, relieves anxiety, treats asthma; and bacterial infections.
- Parts used: flowers
- Preparations/Dosage: Can be eaten raw or brewed into a tea. You can also dry and powder passionflower, make it into syrup, or make a tincture.
- **Caution: Should not be used by pregnant women or before surgery.**

86. Pearly Everlasting

- Scientific name: *Anaphalis margaritacea*
- Other names: Western pearly everlasting
- Description: Perennial plant with narrow, alternating leaves that have hairy undersides. dry, brittle stems. Small yellowish-white flowers grow in clusters and have white bracts.
- Location: Throughout the US
- Medicinal uses: treats sores, rheumatism, and diarrhea.
- Parts used: the whole plant.
- Preparations/Dosage: Create a poultice for sores. Boil in tea to take internally or add to hot, steamy baths for aches.

87. Pecan

- Scientific name: *Carya illinoensis.*
- Description: Pecan trees have large, major limbs that become wide-sweeping with age. The deciduous leaves have serrated margins and grow alternately. The trees produce nuts in the fall.
- Location: Throughout the US
- Season: fall.
- Medicinal uses: improves cardiovascular and brain health.
- Parts used: nuts.
- Preparations/Dosage: Eat raw or roast. You can extract pecan oil.
- **Caution: Avoid if allergic to nuts.**

88. Pine

- Scientific name: *Pinus strobus.*
- Other names: white pine, northern pine.
- Description: A tall, evergreen tree with horizontal branches. produces pale-green needles and drooping, cylindrical pine cones.
- Location: Northern States
- Season: fall.
- Medicinal uses: antimicrobial; fights respiratory infections when used as a rub or internally.
- Parts used: resin and needles.

- Preparations/Dosage: The cones may contain edible nuts. The resin can be applied to the skin as a rub. The needles can be made into tea.
- **Caution: Try not to damage the tree when harvesting resin.**

89. Plantain

- Scientific name: *Plantago.*
- Other names: common plantain, broad-leaved plantain, narrow-leaved plantain.
- Description: A perennial, low-growing herb with a rosette of basal leaves (either broad or narrow). produces a dense flower spike.
- Location: Throughout the US
- Medicinal uses: it heals wounds, fevers, insect bites, and toothaches. Antibacterial qualities.
- Parts used: leaves.
- Preparations/Dosage: Create a poultice for external use, a tincture, or steeped tea to drink.

90.Pleurisy Root

- Scientific name: *Asclepias tuberosa.*
- Other names: butterfly weed
- Description: Bloom has distinctively large umbels of orange, red, or yellow 5-petaled flowers. It has hairy stems that aren't milky when broken.

- Location: Eastern and southwestern US.
- Season: Fall.
- Medicinal uses: Treats diarrhea, bruises, swelling, and respiratory illnesses, like pleurisy.
- Parts used: roots.
- Preparations/Dosage: Boil the roots and eat or drink them as tea. Create a poultice for external use.
- **Caution: Do not use it when pregnant. toxic in large quantities.**

91. Prickly Ash

- Scientific name: *Zanthoxylum americanum*
- Other names: common prickly ash, northern prickly ash, toothache tree
- Description: An aromatic shrub with dark green, pinnately compound leaves and yellow-green flowers that grow in clusters.
- Location: Oklahoma
- Season: fall
- Medicinal uses: antifungal. treats toothaches, colds, inflammation, digestive complaints, and rheumatism.
- Parts used: bark and berries
- Preparations/Dosage: Chew on the bark or make tea by boiling it in water. Tinctures can be made with berries and bark.

92. Prickly Lettuce

- Scientific name: *Lactuca serriola*
- Other names: wild lettuce, lettuce opium.
- Description: Herbaceous plant with solid stems and deeply lobed, clasping leaves that grow alternately. The leaves are often turned sideways for more sun exposure. Produces small, yellow flowers that mature into seedheads.
- Location: Throughout the US.
- Season: Spring.
- Medicinal uses: relieves pain and tension and has a calming effect. Sleep aid.
- Parts used: leaves and stem.
- Preparations/Dosage: Create a fresh plant tincture, and dilute it into drinks.
- **Caution: It may cause drowsiness. Be careful if you have depression or low stomach acid.**

93. Prickly Pear

- Scientific name: *Opuntia*
- Other names: pear cactus
- Description: Segmented cactus with large green or blue-green pads. has large spines and smaller hairs. produces large, spiral-shaped flowers and ovoid, red fruits.
- Location: Western and southern US in desert areas.

- Medicinal uses: treats wounds, inflammation, digestive problems, and urinary issues. Coagulant for wounds.
- Parts used: fruit (pulp and juice)
- Preparations/Dosage: Use pulp as a poultice. Drink the juice.
- **Caution: Watch out for spines and hair.**

94. Prickly Poppy

- Scientific name: *Argemone mexicana.*
- Other names: Mexican poppy, flowering thistle.
- Description: Has small yellow bowl-shaped flowers and thistle-like, sharply toothed, dark green leaves.
- Location: Western US
- Medicinal uses: Treats postnatal kidney pain, acts as a laxative, treats malaria and jaundice.
- Parts used: the whole plant
- Preparations/Dosage: Make an infusion with the fresh or dried plant.
- **Caution: The seeds and oil can be toxic.**

95. Puncture Vine

- Scientific name: *Tribulus terrestris*
- Other names: goat's head, bullhead, tackweed.
- Description: Invasive species that grow in patches. Stems and leaves are hairy. Leaves are pinnately

compound. The yellow flowers mature into fruits that turn into five sharp, hard burs.

- Location: Dry, warm areas throughout the US.
- Medicinal uses: improves heart health, and blood pressure and treats infections, pain, kidney stones, and sexual or reproductive issues.
- Parts used: fruit, leaves, roots.
- Preparations/Dosage: Take as a tincture, 5 ml spread over each day.
- **Caution: Can interact with medications—possible links to prostate problems. Do not take it while pregnant.**

96. Queen's Root

- Scientific name: *Stillingia linearifolia.*
- Description: A perennial herb with slender, erect stems that branch off. The leaves are linear and narrow. The flowers grow on a spike, and the plant produces distinctive green capsules.
- Location: Southwestern US
- Season: fall.
- Medicinal uses Chest problems, piles, skin abscesses, muscle spasms.
- Parts used: root.
- Preparations/Dosage: Create an herbal extract or boil for tea.
- **Caution: It can have side effects.**

97. Red Root

- Scientific name: *Ceanothus americanus*
- Other names: New Jersey tea, mountain sweet, wild snowball.
- Description: Shrubs with many thin branches and white flowers grow in clusters. The roots consist of both fibrous and woody roots
- Location: Throughout the US
- Season: fall
- Medicinal uses: treats upper respiratory tract infections and lymphatic system issues, lowers blood pressure, and is an astringent.
- Parts used: roots and leaves.
- Preparations/Dosage: The red roots and the root bark can be boiled into a tea. The leaves can also be made into a stimulating tea.

98. Rhatany

- Scientific name: *Krameria*.
- Description: Small, perennial shrubs with hairy branches and fuzzy leaves. has a deep taproot. The flowers range in color from pink to red.
- Location: Southwestern US.
- Season: fall.
- Medicinal uses: used as a lozenge or to treat diarrhea or toothache.

- Parts used: roots.
- Preparations/Dosage: Create an infusion to gargle. Roots can be dried and powdered to relieve toothache.

99. Rosemary Mint

- Scientific name: *Poliomintha.*
- Other names: Frosted mint.
- Description: Aromatic shrub with dark green leaves covered in white hairs. Has small purple or blue tubular flowers.
- Location: Southwestern US.
- Medicinal uses: Treats sores, rheumatism, and ear problems.
- Parts used: edible sweet leaves.
- Preparations/Dosage: Create a poultice for external use. It can be added to other medicinal herb mixes for flavor and to increase potency.

100. Sage

- Scientific name: *Salvia officinalis*
- Other names: garden sage, common sage.
- Description: Leafy perennial shrub. The leaves are green, aromatic, and fuzzy.
- Location: Throughout the US.

- Medicinal uses: Digestive aid lowers blood pressure and can improve memory and cognition.
- Parts used: leaves.
- Preparations/Dosage: Eat as an herb, either raw or cooked. It can be used in tea or turned into a tincture for medicinal purposes. Take a few drops of tincture a day.
- **Caution: Pregnant women, people with hypertension, and those who suffer from seizures shouldn't ingest too much sage.**

101. Self-heal

- Scientific name: *Prunella vulgaris*
- Other names: allheall, heal-all.
- Description: A low-growing weed that spreads to cause ground cover. It has square stems and simple leaves, and the stem terminates in a cylindrical cluster of small flowers. See diagram 2 (page 64)
- Location: Throughout the US
- Medicinal uses: anti-inflammatory, antibacterial and support immunity. Treats dizziness, red eyes, cold, cough, dermatitis, throat problems, and boils. Also edible, it can be used for soup, stew, and salad.
- Parts used: The whole plant.
- Preparations/Dosage: Use as herb or create a cold plant infusion, and oxymel

102. Shepherd's Purse

- Scientific name: *Capsella bursa-pastoris*
- Description: An erect stem grows from a rosette of basal lobed leaves. A few pointed leaves grow further up the stem. Blooms small white flowers that produce flattened purse-like seed pods. See diagram 4 (page 66)
- Location: Throughout the US.
- Medicinal uses: Stops bleeding, treats eye problems and dysentery.
- Parts used: leaves.
- Preparations/Dosage: leaves can be eaten raw. You can make a poultice for external use or tea.

103. Siberian Elm

- Scientific name: *Ulmus pumila.*
- Other names: dwarf elm, Asiatic elm.
- Description: A small, bushy, deciduous tree with dark gray, fissured bark. Flowers bloom for one week in early spring before the leaves emerge in bundles.
- Location: Throughout the US.
- Medicinal uses: Diuretic, treats fevers, can treat abscesses, swelling, and mastitis.
- Parts used: leaves, stem bark.

- Preparations/Dosage: leaves can be used as a pot herb or tea. Bark can be made into a poultice.

104. Silk Tassel

- Scientific name: *Garrya.*
- Other names: tassel bush.
- Description: Evergreen shrubs with simple, leathery, dark green, ovate leaves. They produce gray-green pendulous catkins.
- Location: Western US.
- Medicinal Uses: Antispasmodic, treats menstrual cramps, asthma, dysentery, stomach cramps, and coughing fits.
- Parts used: leaves and twigs.
- Preparations/Dosage: Make a tincture from dried leaves and twigs or an extract with the fresh leaves.

105. Skullcap

- Scientific name: *Scutellaria lateriflora*
- Other names: blue skullcap, American skullcap.
- Description: upright plant with branches. Produces small bluish purple flowers on the side branches that grow from leaf axils.
- Location: Wetlands throughout the US.
- Medicinal uses: as a sedative, treats anxiety and inflammation, and can regulate menstruation.

- Parts used: leaves
- Preparations/Dosage: Dry leaves for tea or make a tincture and take a few drops to induce sleep.
- **Caution: Do not use it when pregnant.**

106. Snakeweed

- Scientific name: *Gutierrezia.*
- Other names: matchweeds.
- Description: Heavily branched shrub. Old parts are brown and woody, while new shoots are green or yellow. Leaves are threadlike. produces small clusters of yellow flowers.
- Location: Species found throughout Western and Southern US, usually in arid or desert areas.
- Medicinal uses: treats toothache, acts as a diuretic and tonic, and induces sweating.
- Parts used: flowers
- Preparations/Dosage: Create an infusion for gargling or steep flower heads in boiling water for tea. can create a poultice.
- **Caution: Toxic to livestock. Do not use it when pregnant.**

107. Sow Thistle

- Scientific name: *Sonchus*
- Other names: hare thistles, hair lettuce.

- Description: Herb with soft, irregularly lobed leaves that form a basal rosette. The stem contains milky latex. grows small yellow ray flowers. It looks similar to dandelions.
- Location: Throughout the US.
- Medicinal uses: Treats headaches, pain, diarrhea, menstrual issues, fever, warts, infections, and inflammation.
- Parts used: the whole plant.
- Preparations/Dosage: sap from stems can be used to treat warts. Leaves can be made into a poultice or cleansing juice. You can also cook and eat stems and leaves. Create an infusion to drink. A decoction of a plant can make an ointment.

108. Spanish Needle

- Scientific name: *Bidens bipinnata.*
- Description: An annual herb with heavily toothed leaves and erect, branching stems. produces white or yellow flower heads, including disk and ray florets.
- Location: throughout the US.
- Medicinal uses: Treats asthma and lung issues, as well as sore throats, boils, and wounds.
- Parts used: the whole plant
- Preparations/Dosage: Chew leaves for sore throat. Warm leaf juice can be used topically. Create a tincture from the whole plant.

109. Spiderwort

- Scientific Name: *Tradescantia virginiana.*
- Other names: inchplant, dayflower.
- Description: Herbaceous perennials with tubular stems and alternate, simple leaves. Blue, purple, magenta, or white 3-petaled flowers bloom in the summer.
- Location: Texas, Arizona.
- Season: fall.
- Medicinal uses: laxative; treats period pain, kidney and stomach issues, stings, and minor wounds.
- Parts used: Roots and leaves
- Preparations/Dosage: Create a root decoction for a laxative. The leaves can be made into tea or a poultice for external use.

110. Spikenard

- Scientific name: *Aralia racemosa.*
- Other names: American spikenard, Indian root, petty morel, spice berry.
- Description: Herbaceous plant with broad, toothed compound leaves that bears clusters of purple-red fruits in the fall.
- Location: eastern US.
- Season: fall.

- Medicinal uses: Treats coughs, colds, menstrual problems, kidney problems, burns, wounds, swelling, sprains, and broken bones.
- Parts used: Roots
- Preparations/Dosage: Create a root infusion for internal use. Apply a poultice for external use.

111. Sweet Clover

- Scientific name: *Melilotus officinalis*
- Other names: melilot, sweet yellow clover.
- Description: A tall plant with an erect stem and alternate, triple compound leaves. The stems terminate in a tall cluster of yellow, drooping flowers. has a sweet smell.
- Location: Invasive throughout the US.
- Season: spring and summer.
- Medicinal uses: Treats sleeplessness, neuralgia, palpitations, menstrual cramps, intestinal issues, swollen joints, boils, eye infections, and skin infections.
- Parts used: flowering tops.
- Preparations/Dosage: A flower infusion can be used as an eye wash or drink. Create a decoction and add it to bath water for external use.
- **Caution: Anticoagulants can interfere with blood disorders.**

112. Thistle

- Scientific name: *Cirsium vulgare*
- Other names: common thistle, spear thistle, bull thistle.
- Description: A tall plant with a rosette of leaves and a long taproot. It forms a flowering stem with spiny wings and is topped with a pinkish-purple inflorescence. forms downy seeds.
- Location: Throughout the US
- Medicinal uses: diuretic; treats liver problems, fever, stiff neck, soreness, and nervous disorders.
- Parts used: leaves and roots
- Preparations/Dosage: A poultice of leaves and roots can be applied to sore areas. The boiled leaves can be drunk.

113. Tickseed

- Scientific name: *Coreopsis tinctoria*
- Other names: plains coreopsis, garden tickseed.
- Description: This plant has pinnately divided leaves that thin further up the plant. has slender stems that support yellow flower heads with brown or maroon disc florets.
- Location: Throughout the US.
- Season: fall.

- Medicinal uses: emetic, treats diarrhea, pain, and bleeding.
- Parts used: roots
- Preparations/Dosage: Boil roots for tea.

114. Tree of Heaven

- Scientific name: *Ailanthus altissima*
- Other names: varnish tree, ailanthus.
- Description: A medium tree with smooth, gray bark and reddish or brown twigs. Leaves are pinnately compound on the stem. The small flowers grow in clusters and are yellowish-green or reddish. They mature into reddish-brown fruits.
- Location: Invasive throughout the US.
- Season: fall.
- Medicinal uses: Treats fever, gastric diseases, inflammation, asthma, cramps, and diarrhea.
- Parts used: root and bark.
- Preparations/Dosage: Dry the root or bark and boil for tea.
- **Caution: It may be mildly toxic, with noxious odors when burnt.**

115. Velvet Mesquite

- Scientific name: *Prosopis velutina*

- Description: A small tree with reddish-brown bark that matures into a rugged gray color. grows inch-long yellow thorns on the branches. The leaves are long and fold at night.
- Location: Arizona.
- Season: fall.
- Medicinal uses: sore throat, stomach ache, toothache, helps appetite.
- Parts used: sap, inner red bark, root bark, leaves.
- Preparations/Dosage: You can make tea with sap bark or fresh leaves. Chew soft roots for toothache.

116. Violet

- Scientific Name: *Viola*
- Description: Herbs with short stems, simple kidney-shaped leaves, and 5-petaled flowers. The flowers are often violet in color but may have other colors.
- Location: Throughout the US.
- Medicinal uses: A sleep aid treats inflammation, skin irritation, and swelling.
- Parts used: flowers and leaves.
- Preparations/Dosage: Make into a tea or a soothing poultice.

117. Walnut

- Scientific name: *Juglans regia*

- Description: Deciduous tree with either brown or gray bark. Walnuts grow in bunches of 3 to 9 and fall from the tree when ripe.
- Location: Throughout the US
- Season: fall.
- Medicinal uses: lowers cholesterol, protects the heart, and fights infection.
- Parts used: nuts and leaves.
- Preparations/Dosage: Eat as snacks. Leaves and nuts can be brewed into a tea or macerated and made into a tincture. Walnut oil can be rubbed into the skin.
- **Caution: Avoid if allergic to nuts.**

118. Western Peony

- Scientific name: *Paeonia brownii*
- Other names: Brown's peony, native peony
- Description: Herbaceous plant with up to 10 pinkish stems per plant, each growing from a large, fleshy root. grows blueish-green fleshy leaves. The flowers are cup-shaped and nod.
- Location: Western US.
- Season: fall.
- Medicinal uses: Treats lung conditions, kidney problems, nausea, and indigestion.
- Parts used: root.
- Preparations/Dosage: Boil into a tea.

119. Wild Buckwheat

- Scientific name: *Eriogonum*
- Description: Forms a shrub or mat with long, narrow leaves. The tiny flowers are either pink or white and grow in dense clusters.
- Location: Species found throughout the US.
- Medicinal uses: Treats headaches, diarrhea, sore throats, and wounds.
- Parts used: leaves, stems, and roots.
- Preparations/Dosage: It can be made into a tea to be taken internally. A root poultice or decoction can treat wounds. The decoction can also be drunk.

120. Wild Mint

- Scientific name: *Mentha arvensis*
- Other names: corn mint, field mint.
- Description: Herbaceous plant with erect or semi-sprawling square stems. The broad, hairy leaves grow in opposite pairs. produces small pale purple flowers in whorls at the base of the leaves.
- Location: Temperate regions of the US.
- Medicinal uses: aids digestion and treats colds.
- Parts used: leaves
- Preparations/Dosage: Eat it raw or make it into tea.

121. Wild Oregano

- Scientific name: Origanum vulgare
- Other names: wild marjoram.
- Description: A perennial herb with spade-shaped green leaves and small purple funnel-shaped flowers.
- Location: throughout the US.
- Season: summer.
- Medicinal uses: Treats coughs and wounds, aids digestion, and fights infections.
- Parts used: leaves
- Preparations/Dosage: Can be used as an herb. It can be used to create essential oils.

122. Wild Tobacco

- Scientific name: *Nicotiana obtusifolia*
- Other names: desert tobacco.
- Description: A woody herb with lower leaves on petioles and smaller upper leaves attached to the stem. produces white funnel-shaped flowers.
- Location: California, Utah, and Texas
- Medicinal uses: Treats rheumatic or painful swelling and skin problems.
- Parts used: leaves
- Preparations/Dosage: Create a poultice or decoction to use externally.
- **Caution: It contains nicotine.**

123. Willow Tree (Black)

- Scientific name: *Salix nigra*
- Description: A fast-growing deciduous tree, 10–60 ft. tall, with an open crown and several trunks growing out at angles from one root. Alternate, simple, 5-inch long blade leaves, Bright yellow-green twigs bear yellow catkins. The barks are deeply furrowed.
- Location: Texas (native), Oklahoma, New Mexico
- Season: summer.
- Medicinal uses: rheumatism, gout, fever, cough, headache, and poultice for cuts,wounds,sprains, and bruises.
- Parts used: leaves, and bark
- Preparations/Dosage: bark tincture, infusion , poultice
- **Caution: Avoid allergic salicin (aspirin), children under age 16, pregnancy, and breastfeeding. It also interacts with some medications, such as blood thinners and diuretics.**

124. Yarrow

- Scientific Name: *Achillea milifolium*
- Other names: common yarrow, milfoil, soldier's woundwort.

- Description: Erect a plant with one or more stems and evenly distributed feathery leaves arranged spirally on the stems. produces clusters of white or pink flowers.
- Location: temperate areas in the US.
- Medicinal uses: astringent, laxative, treating toothaches, earaches, colds, pain, fevers, and healing cuts.
- Parts used: leaves.
- Preparations/Dosage: Create an infused or steeped tea with the leaves, or chew for toothaches. Make a poultice for external use.
- **Caution: Do not ingest when pregnant. toxic to some animals.**

125. Yerba Mansa

- Scientific name: *Anemopsis*
- Other names: lizard tail
- Description: Blooms distinctive white flower clusters with large white bracts that look like petals. As the leaves mature, they turn red. grows in marshes.
- Location: Southwestern US.
- Medicinal uses: antimicrobial, antifungal, diuretic, and anti-inflammatory. treats wounds and sores.
- Parts used: roots and leaves
- Preparations/Dosage: Take orally as a tea, tincture, or infusion. The leaves can be used as a poultice. The

dried powder can be taken in capsules or used externally for fungal infections.

126. Yerba Santa

- Scientific name: *Eriodictyon angustifolium*
- Other names: narrowleaf yerba santa, holy herb, mountain balm.
- Description: A perennial shrub with toothed, long leaves that are sticky and hairy underneath. Blooms white, 5-petaled flowers in summer.
- Location: California, Southwestern US
- Medicinal uses: treats cough, asthma, rheumatism, wounds, bites, sores, and broken bones. It can reduce graying.
- Parts used: leaves
- Preparations/Dosage: Create a tea for internal use or a poultice for external use.

127. Yucca

- Scientific name: *Yucca angustissima*
- Other names: narrowleaf Yucca
- Description: Forms colonies of basal rosettes with long, thin leaves. produces white-ish flowers in clusters on stalks up to 7 feet tall. fruits into a dry capsule.

- Location: California, New Mexico, Texas, Arizona, Colorado
- Medicinal uses: antiemetic, prevents vomiting. Laxative.
- Parts used: leaves
- Preparations/Dosage: Create infusion with leaves

Now that we have explored the 127 medicinal plants you can find across the United States, the next chapter explains how to convert weights and measures from the imperial system to the metric system and vice versa.

Medicinal Plants profile photos QR code

METRIC CONVERSIONS

As well as learning how to harvest medicinal herbs safely, you must also understand how to accurately measure ingredients for processing your herbs and preparing medicines. If you're based in the US, you're likely familiar with culinary measurements, such as teaspoons, tablespoons, cups, and imperial weights. However, herbal recipes use different measurements.

VOLUME VS. WEIGHT

In the US, most culinary recipes use volume and the imperial measurement system. When you're weighing something that is liquid or has a uniform shape, such as water or flour, weighing by volume is relatively accurate.

Because it is so important to accurately measure ingredients for herbal medicines, most herbal recipes use weight instead of volume to ensure that you use the same amount of medicinal plants every time. However, measuring by volume is no longer accurate when weighing ingredients that don't have a uniform shape, like herbs or other medicinal plant parts. For example, if you put whole curly dock leaves into one cup and chopped leaves into another, both cups will hold different amounts of herbs. Measuring by weight can also be more straightforward. You can't simply fill a tablespoon of the ingredient, but once you have a set of accurate scales and get used to using them, measuring by weight is reliable and easy.

When measuring your ingredients, it's vital to stick to one measurement system. If you change the units around, it's easy to get confused and measure out too much of one ingredient. An ounce is about 28 times heavier than a gram, which means that if you mix up these units, you could make something much bigger than you meant. This is another advantage of using weights over volume, especially if you're using an international recipe. In the US, a tablespoon of water is 15 ml, while in Australia, a tablespoon measures 20 ml. However, a gram is the same worldwide.

PRACTICAL MEASUREMENTS

Depending on what kind of medicinal preparation you make, you might not need to be too precise with your measurements. For example, if you're making a pot of herbal tea, there's nothing wrong with measuring ingredients for processing your herbs and preparing medicines accurately. Share a tea blend recipe; you will need to measure the ingredients. Herbal tea involves low doses of diluted medicinal plants so that you can be more relaxed. This is especially true once you become more familiar with making tea blends and develop experience and intuition for what works.

Also, some medicinal preparation methods require accurate measuring, no matter how experienced you are. Tincture formulas, herbal and essential oils, and liniments should all be carefully weighed.

OUNCES VS. GRAMS

The Imperial Measurement System, primarily used in the US, uses measurements like inches, ounces, and pounds. However, the metric system is generally suited for measuring small amounts of medicinal plant parts, giving you more precise measurements. Measuring 5 grams of chicory root for a tincture is far easier than 0.176 ounces. Herbal recipes will use grams.

PARTS VS. RATIO

Many herbal recipes involve measuring in parts or by ratio. Measuring in parts allows you to better control the strength of tinctures, extracts, oils, and other herbal preparations. For example, a fresh alcohol tincture consists of 1 part of fresh ingredients and two parts of alcohol. If you have 50 grams of fresh ingredients, you will need 100 grams (or ml) of alcohol. But if you have 500 grams of fresh ingredients, you know to stick to the same ratio and use 1000 ml of alcohol. By measuring in parts, you can make batches of different sizes and still end up with the same result, which means that you can accurately measure out dosages.

CONCLUSION

GLOSSARY OF FORAGING TERMS

- Aerial Parts: A plant's parts that grow above ground.
- Alternate Leaves: Leaf arrangement where they grow singly at nodes and not as opposite pairs.
- Basal: The base of a plant, leaves that grow at ground level.
- Bloom: Developmental stage where the plant grows flowers.
- Bracts: A modified leaf that grows at the base of a flower/inflorescence.
- Bulb: An underground storage organ akin to a seed.
- Compound leaf: A leaf composed of at least two similar parts, known as leaflets.

- Coniferous: A group of evergreen cone-bearing seed plants.
- Deciduous: Perennial woody plants that lose their leaves in winter.
- Evergreen: Keeps green leaves throughout the year.
- Fibrous: Root system with many fine branches.
- Flower: The sexual reproductive structure of a plant, typically consisting of petals and male/female sexual organs.
- Fruit: The ripened ovary of a plant typically carries the seeds.
- Habitat: The living place of an organism or community.
- Herbicide: Chemicals designed to kill plants.
- Inflorescence: Flowering structure composed of multiple flowers.
- Invasive: A species introduced to an area and replaced native plants to the detriment of the ecosystem.
- Margin: The outer edge of a leaf or other structure.
- Mature: A plant that grows flowers and can reproduce sexually.
- Native: A species that occurs naturally in an area and that hasn't been introduced by humans.
- Naturalized: A species initially imported from another country and now behaves like a native. It may or may not be detrimental.
- Node: The place where a leaf joins the stem.

- Perennial: A plant that lives for more than two seasons and produces flowers annually.
- Sap: The fluid that forms from the wounded tissue of a plant.
- Serrate: Sharp teeth that point forwards, like a saw blade. Used to describe leaf margins.
- Simple leaf: A leaf not divided into leaflets.
- Spike: An unbranched inflorescence.
- Taproot: A primary descending root.
- Tuber: Storage organs in the dormant season form on the roots of some leafy plants.
- Vegetative: A structure or stage concerned with feeding and growth, leaves are vegetative.

GLOSSARY OF HERBALTERMS

- Analgesic: Substance that relieves pain.
- Antibiotic: Inhibits growth of bacteria.
- Anti-inflammatory: Reduces inflammation.
- Antiseptic: A substance that inhibits the growth of microorganisms and prevents decay.
- Astringent: Substances that contract tissues and regulate body secretions.
- Compress: Cloth or gauze soaked in a liquid herbal preparation applied externally to the body.
- Decoction: A concentrated water extraction of plant material made by boiling the plant part for an extended time.

- Decongestant: Substance that relieves congestion.
- Diuretic: Substance that promotes the production and expulsion of urine.
- Emetic: Substance that induces vomiting.
- Expectorant: Substance that loosens mucus, allowing it to be coughed up.
- Herbal Medicine: The medicinal use of plants to treat disease and support general health.
- Infusion: A drink made by soaking the plant in hot or cold water.
- Infused Oil: An oil that results from soaking the plant in oil.
- Laxative: A substance that promotes bowel evacuation.
- Poultice: A soft, moist mixture of plant material applied topically.
- Salve: A semi-solid, fatty herbal mixture applied topically.
- Sedative: A substance that promotes sleep and relaxation.
- Tincture: A concentrated plant extract made by soaking the plant material in a medium, such as glycerin, alcohol, or vinegar.
- Tonic: A substance that stimulates and energizes the body.

FINAL THOUGHTS

The Southwestern United States holds plenty of medicinal herbs to find and use. All you need to do is get out there and explore the wide variety of habitats to discover what they have to offer. Whether you take to the wilderness or stick to green spots in urban areas, you will find a bounty of goodness waiting for you. However, always remember to forage responsibly. Take only what you need, make sure not to overharvest or damage the ecosystem, and if you need to, ask permission. This way, you can continue to enjoy the medicinal herbs that nature has to offer.

Foraging for medicinal plants is a massive part of my life and how I keep myself and my family healthy. If you're responsible, you can take full advantage of nature's potential to improve your well-being. I hope that this guide will be a helpful and informative companion on your way to making medicine, and that it will help you see nature in a new way.

Share the Knowledge!

It used to be that knowledge about plants and foraging was passed down through stories and skill-sharing... Now we have to take matters into our own hands... and I need your help.

Simply by sharing your honest opinion of this book on Amazon, you'll show new readers where they can find everything they need to know to start foraging for medicinal plants.

LEAVE A REVIEW!

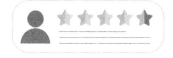

Thank you for your support. Together, we can bring this essential knowledge back into common understanding.

Scan this QR code to leave your review!

RESOURCES

INTRODUCTION AND CHAPTER 1

Žarko Šantić, Nikolina Pravdić, Milenko Bevanda & Kristina Galić (2017).The historical use of medicinal plants in traditional and scientific medicine.
Psychiatria Danubina, 2017; Vol. 29, Suppl. 4, pp S787–S792 Medicina Academica Mostariensia, 2017; Vol. 5, No. 1-2, pp 69-74 Review © Medicinska naklada - Zagreb, Croatia
https://www.psychiatria-danubina.com/UserDocsImages/pdf/dnb_vol29%20Suppl%204/dnb_vol29%20Suppl%204_noSuppl%204_69.pdf
Tibi Puiu (2021). Medicinal plant extract used by native Americans treats both pain and diarrhea.
ZMEScience.com.Health & medicine, News 2021
https://www.zmescience.com/science/news-science/medicinal-plant-extract-used-by-native-americans-can-treat-both-pain-and-diarrhea/
Shurkin, J. (2014, December 9). *Animals that self-medicate*. Pnas.org.
https://www.pnas.org/doi/10.1073/pnas.1419966111
Akinyemi O, Oyewole SO, Jimoh KA.(2018) Medicinal plants and sustainable human health: a review.
Horticult Int J. 2018;2(4):194-195.
https://medcraveonline.com/HIJ/medicinal-plants-and-sustainable-human-health-a-review.html
Beth Judy. (2021) Nature is medicine.
Ask a biologist, Arizona State University.26.10. 2010
https://askabiologist.asu.edu/explore/natures-medicine Sa
Sarah Garone. (2020) What is wild food and should you do eating?
VerywellFit.com 04.06.2020
https://www.verywellfit.com/what-is-wild-food-4797692
Daniijela Grizelji, MSc(2020)The importance of plants in the pharmaceutical industry.
Martifarm.com 15.10.2020

https://martifarm.com/the-importance-of-plants-in-the-pharmaceutical-industry/

Beth Judy. (2021) Nature is medicine.

Ask a biologist, Arizona State University. 26.10. 2010

https://askabiologist.asu.edu/medicinal-plants

Herbal medicine. (2021)

betterhealth.vi.go.au

https://www.betterhealth.vic.gov.au/health/conditionsandtreatments/herbal-medicine

WTHN team. (2020) The Benefit of Herbal Medicine: Power of Plants.

Wthn.com blog.

https://wthn.com/blogs/wthnside-out/the-benefits-of-herbal-medicine-power-of-plants

Rob Greenfield.21.03.2020.The database to find a forager near you!

Findforager.com

https://www.robgreenfield.org/findaforager

CHAPTER 2

Julie Douglas. (2021)Ethical Foraging-Responsibility and Reciprocity.

Organic Growers School. 06.05.2021

https://organicgrowersschool.org/ethical-foraging-responsibility-and-reciprocity/

Tree principles for Ethical foraging.

The Druids Garden blog. 16.04.2022

https://druidgarden.wordpress.com/2021/08/15/three-principles-for-an-ethical-foraging-practice-harvest-mindfully-tend-the-wilds-and-build-knowledge/

Devon Young (20.03.2017) Ethical foraging 101: What to need to know.

Gardening and skills.

https://learningherbs.com/skills/foraging/

Foraging wild food.

Edible Wild Food. (2021)

https://www.ediblewildfood.com/foraging-for-food.aspx

Sam Sycamore. Seven rules of foraging; Read this before gathering wild foods.

Good life reveals blog. March.30
https://thegoodliferevival.com/blog/foraging-rules

CHAPTER 3

How to Identify poisonous plants in the garden.
Balcon Garden Web.2021
https://balconygardenweb.com/how-to-identify-poisonous-plants-in-the-garden/
Kelly Hodgkins(2021) Poisonous Plants Identification Guide.
Green belly Website. Updated on 10.04.2021.
https://www.greenbelly.co/pages/poisonous-plants-identification-guide
Common poisonous plants and plant parts.
Earth-Kind Landscaping, Texas A&M University System
https://aggie-horticulture.tamu.edu/earthkind/landscape/poisonous-plants-resources/common-poisonous-plants-and-plant-parts/
Katy Licavoli. (26.05.2021) A guide using The Universal Edibility Test using to identify poisonous plants.
The Universal Edibility Test, Green belly website
https://www.greenbelly.co/pages/universal-edibility-test
Scott Sexton. (2021) How to not die while wildcrafting; 15 rules for foraging safely.
Grow network website.27.08.2021
https://thegrownetwork.com/wildcrafting-foraging-safely/
International Culinary Center(2018) How to safely forage.
Institute of Culinary Education.28.11.2018
https://www.ice.edu/blog/how-to-safely-forage
Paul Skidmore. (2021) Best foraging accessories in 2021.
Mountain website..17.08.2021
https://mountain.co.uk/best-foraging-accessories-in-2021
Kevin Estella and AGS staff. Foraging gear: Tools you need to collect, process, and carry natural food.
American outdoor guide. Boundless.22.03.2018.
https://www.americanoutdoor.guide/how-to/foraging-gear-the-tools-you-need-to-collect-process-and-carry-natural-foods/

Thordur Sturluson. (2017) Ethical foraging; Do and Don'ts
The Herbal Resource. 03.04.2017.
https://www.herbal-supplement-resource.com/ethical-foraging/
Trent Blizzard. (03.04.2018) The best GPSApp for mushroom hunting: Gaya GPS
Modern forager website.
https://www.modern-forager.com/the-best-gps-app-for-mushroom-hunt ing-gaia-gps/
CBS news.(*03.04.*2011). Giant hogweed: 8 facts you must know about toxic plants.
CBS news website.
https://www.cbsnews.com/pictures/giant-hogweed-8-facts-you-must-know-about-the-toxic-plan
Getwell Urgent Care. (07.02.2020) Southern Discomfort: A Complete to the Mid-South's Most Poisonous Plants.
Blog: Health news from Getwell Urgent Care
https://urgentcaresouthaven.com/southern-discomfort-a-complete-guide-to-the-mid-souths-most-poisonous-plants/
How to Identify Poisonous Plants - Emergency Essentials." 17 Jun. 2014, https://beprepared.com/blogs/articles/how-to-identify-poisonous-plants. Accessed 17 Apr. 2023.
Poisonous Plants: Symptoms and First Aid
May 24, 2022.National Institute for Occupational Safety and Health
https://www.cdc.gov/niosh/topics/plants/symptoms.html

CHAPTER4,5

Thomas J.Elpel. (2021) Plants of The Pea Family.
Wildflowers-and-Weeds.com.Web World Portal (1997-2021)
https://www.wildflowers-and-weeds.com/Plant_Families/Fabaceae.htm
Tayler Jenkins.Greg.(11.11,2013) Edible and Medicinal Plants of the Desert Southwest.
The Urban Farm. A Blog Article
Edible and Medicinal Plants of the Desert Southwest - The Urban Farm
Jamie Nielson, Kelly Reeves, and Lisa Thomas,(2010) Grassland of the

American Southwest-Introduction and Grassland Types

National Park Service.Southern Colorado Plateau Network Inventory and Monitoring Program,

www.nps.gov/articles/southwest-grasslands.htm

By admin. (*28.02.*2015) Arizona National Parks List

National Park.com.

https://www.national-park.com/arizona-national-parks-list/.

T. Beth Kinsey(2022) Edible plants.

Southeastern Arizona Wildflowers and Plants. fireflyforest.com

https://www.fireflyforest.com/flowers/category/edible-plants/

The Plant List. Helping you find the perfect native plant for your landscape.

The Arizona Native Plant Society. 2022

https://aznps.com/the-plant-list/

Griffith G, E, Omernik, J.M.Johnson, C.B, and Turner, DS, (2014) Ecoregions of Arizona (poster)

US Geological Survey Open-File Report 2014-1141,

https://pubs.usgs.gov/of/2014/1141/pdf/ofr2014-1141_front.pdf

Grand Canyon, National Park Arizona

National Park Service Government website, updated 2022.

https://www.nps.gov/grca/index.htm

Michelle Jacobson(.*01.03.*2016). Foraging in Southern California: Call of the wild.

Edible Orange County web.

California restricts foraging in state parks

BaylenJ. Linnekin(2018). Food Law Gone Wild: The Law of Foraging.

Fordham Urban Law Journal. Vol 45. 995.2018

https://ir.lawnet.fordham.edu/cgi/viewcontent.cgi?article=2740&context=ulj

Kristofor Husted. (23.04.2013) Want to Forage in your city? There's A Map For That.

NPR.The Salt, what is on your plate.23.04. 2013.

https://www.npr.org/sections/thesalt/2013/04/23/178603623/want-to-forage-in-your-city-theres-a-map-for-that

Fallingfruit.org.

Preservation of natural, cultural, and archeological resources.

eCode of Federal Regulations. Title 36. 09.01.2022.

eCFR:: 36 CFR 2.1 -- Preservation of natural, cultural, and archeological resources.

Climate of the Southwestern United States - Earth@Home." 1 Jul. 2022, https://earthathome.org/hoe/sw/climate/. Accessed 18 Apr. 2023.

Climate and Average Weather Year Round in Nevada

Weather Spark website.

https://weatherspark.com/y/9785/Average-Weather-in-Nevada-Missouri-United-States-Year-Round

Colorado rare plant conservation strategy." Colorado rare plant conservation strategy." https://www.conservationgateway.org/ConservationByGeography/NorthAmerica/UnitedStates/Colorado/Documents/CO%20Plant%20Conservation%20Strategy%20Final%20Draft%20march2009.pdf Accessed 18 Apr. 2023.

Colorado Rare Plant Conservation Strategy." 8 Apr. 2009, http://www.cnhp.colostate.edu/download/documents/2009/CO_Plant_Conservation_Strategy_Report-links.pdf. Accessed 18 Apr. 2023.

Edward Franklin Castetter. (2013) Uncultivated native plants used as sources of food

UMN Digital Repository.UMN Bulletins.Scholarly Communication-Departments. 1935

https://digitalrepository.unm.edu/cgi/viewcontent.cgi?article=1022&context=unm_bulletin

Emily Hill(17.01.2018) Finding Healing in New Mexico's Wild Harvest.

Edible New Mexico.Foraged Earth.

https://www.ediblenm.com/foraged-earth/

Griffith G, E, Omernik, McGraw, M M, Jacobi. G.Z (2006) Ecoregion of New Mexico.

Reston Virginia US, Geological Survey(color poster with map, descriptive texts, summary texts, and photographs)

http://ecologicalregions.info/data/nm/nm_front.pdf

Climate of the Southwestern United States - Earth@Home." 1 Jul. 2022, https://earthathome.org/hoe/sw/climate/. Accessed 18 Apr. 2023.

Native Plants. Protected Arizona Native Plants.

Arizona Department of Agriculture website .2022

https://agriculture.az.gov/plantsproduce/native-plants

Elizabeth J. Hermsen, Jonathan R. Hendricks, and Ingrid Zabel in 2022.The climate of the Southwestern US.

Earth@Home website.Paleontological Research Institution.2022
https://earthathome.org/hoe/sw/climate/
Jane Bothwell, March 2000, Analog List for At-Risk and To-Watch Herbs
Species At-Risk List
United Plant Savers
https://unitedplantsavers.org/species-at-risk-list/
50 best sharing knowledge quotes - Words of great wisdom. (2017, May 15).
Quotespeak. https://www.quotespeak.com/professional-quotes/business-quotes/
best-sharing-knowledge-quotes-inspirational-motivational/

CHAPTER 6

Joe Boni.22.11.2021. Nature is beauty and Lessons Within.
Blue Angel House website.
https://blueangelhouse.ca/2021/11/natures-beauty-and-the-lessons-within/
Maria Noel Groves. When and How To Harvest Herbs for Medicinal Use
Storey website, Health & well-being.
https://www.storey.com/article/harvest-herbs-medicinal-use/

CHAPTER 7

Katie Lapsevic. 27.04.2018.How to clean foraged plants.
Homespun Seasonal Living website.
https://homespunseasonalliving.com/clean-foraged-plant
Kristen.Drying. (23.02.2022)
herbs in an air fryer (Quick dehydration method)
Shisandra & Bergamot web.
https://schisandraandbergamot.com/drying-herbs-in-air-fryer/
Emily Nealley. How to dry herbs.
Alderleaf, Wilderness College.
https://www.wildernesscollege.com/how-to-dry-herbs.html
Catherine Winter.Infusion, Decoction, or Tincture? Which Herbal
    Preparations To Use for Different Plant Parts.
Morning Chores website.

https://morningchores.com/herbal-preparations/

Irene. (*20.09.2012*) Herbal Liniments.

Mountain rose herbs.

https://blog.mountainroseherbs.com/making-herbal-liniments

Mary H.Dyer.Using Healing herbs-How to make a Homemade poultice for Healing.

Gardening know-how.

https://www.gardeningknowhow.com/edible/herbs/hgen/homemade-poultice-for-healing.htm

Better health channel, Herbal medicine.

https://www.betterhealth.vic.gov.au/health/conditionsandtreatments/herbal-medicine#bhc-content

PART II PLANTS PROFILE

John Slattery (04.02.2020) Southwest Medicinal Plants: Identify, Harvest, and Use. 112 Wild Herbs for Health and Wellness.

Amazon, Kindle, ebook

My Book

A Nancy, A Praavena. Argemone Mexicana: Boon to Medicinal and Pharmacological Approaches in Current Scenario

Cardiovasc Hematol Agents Med Chem. 30.08.2017 Pubmed.gov National Library of Medicine.

https://www.ncbi.nlm.nih.gov/pmc/articles/PMC6359306/#:~:text=is%20also%20give

American Botanical Council: Food as Medicine update Chia

HerbalEgram,Number 3, March 2020

https://www.herbalgram.org/resources/herbalegram/volumes/volume-17/number-3-march-2020/food-as-medicine-update-chia/food-as-medicine-update-chia/

The American Southwest: Plants of Southwest US

https://www.americansouthwest.net/plants/index.html

GLOSSARY

A-Z Foraging Foraging Glossary. The Language of Plants
Wild plants guide.UK foraging resources and wild plant identification guides.
https://wildplantguides.com/foraging-glossary/
Department of Plants Sciences. A glossary in terms used in Forage identification site.
U.W.Forage Identification-Glossary
http://www.uwyo.edu/plantsciences/uwplant/forages/glossary.html
A-Z Glossary of terms used in herbal medicine. Herbal Glossary of Terms
The Complementary Medical Association
https://www.the-cma.org.uk/articles/az-glossary-of-terms-used-in-herbal-medicine-a-3325/

TABLE CONVERSION -METRIC

Rosalee de la Foret. Making Sense of Herbal Measurements
Herbs with Rosalee
https://www.herbalremediesadvice.org/herbal-measurements.html
Dosage calculations and extract equivalency in herbal medicine.
Ian Breakspear Blog 14.09.2014
https://ianbreakspear.com.au/2014/09/14/dosage-calculations-extract-equivalency-in-herbal-medicine/
Tablespoon Conversions
Conversion-Metric
https://www.conversion-metric.org/volume/tablespoon-conversions

PHOTOS AND ILLUSTRATIONS

127 medicinal plants profile, pixabay.com
inaturalist.org
https://www.inaturalist.org/observations
Illustrations: Diagrams 1-6 (page #) by meow777 Fiverr

NOTES

INTRODUCTION

1. "News Feature: Animals that self-medicate - PMC - NCBI." 9 Dec. 2014, https://www.ncbi.nlm.nih.gov/pmc/articles/PMC4267359/. Accessed 6 Jan. 2023.

1. AN INTRODUCTION TO WILD MEDICINAL PLANTS

1. "Natural products derived from plants as a source of drugs - NCBI." https://www.ncbi.nlm.nih.gov/pmc/articles/PMC3560124/. Accessed 20 Apr. 2023.
2. "Bioactive Non-Nutrients - an overview | ScienceDirect Topics." https://www.sciencedirect.com/topics/food-science/bioactive-non-nutrients. Accessed 20 Apr. 2023.
3. "The discovery of artemisinin and Nobel Prize in Physiology ... - NCBI." 29 Jul. 2016, https://www.ncbi.nlm.nih.gov/pmc/articles/PMC4966551/. Accessed 20 Apr. 2023.

2. GUIDELINES FOR ETHICAL AND SUSTAINABLE FORAGING

1. "22229 UpS Species At-Risk List 2022 rev 7-22 - United Plant Savers." https://unitedplantsavers.org/wp-content/uploads/2022/07/22229-UpS-Species-At-Risk-List-2022-rev-7-22.pdf. Accessed 26 Jan. 2023.

3. SAFETY CONSIDERATIONS WHEN FORAGING

1. "How to Identify Poisonous Plants - Emergency Essentials." 17 Jun. 2014, https://beprepared.com/blogs/articles/how-to-identify-poisonous-plants. Accessed 17 Apr. 2023.

5. LAWS AND LANDS

1. "Promotion of in situ Forest Farmed American Ginseng (Panax ...." 22 Feb. 2021, https://www.frontiersin.org/articles/10.3389/fevo.2021.652103/full. Accessed 21 Apr. 2023.
2. "Climate of the Southwestern United States - Earth@Home." 1 Jul. 2022, https://earthathome.org/hoe/sw/climate/. Accessed 18 Apr. 2023.
3. "colorado rare plant conservation strategy." https://www.conservation gateway.org/ConservationByGeography/NorthAmerica/UnitedStates/Colorado/Documents/CO%20Plant%20Conservation%20Strategy%20Final%20Draft%20march%201%202009.pdf. Accessed 18 Apr. 2023.
4. "Colorado Rare Plant Conservation Strategy." 8 Apr. 2009, http://www.cnhp.colostate.edu/download/documents/2009/CO_Plant_Conservation_Strategy_Report-links.pdf. Accessed 18 Apr. 2023.
5. "Climate of the Southwestern United States - Earth@Home." 1 Jul. 2022, https://earthathome.org/hoe/sw/climate/. Accessed 18 Apr. 2023.

7. MEDICINAL PLANT PREPARATION TECHNIQUES

1. "3 Ways to Make Liniment - wikiHow." https://www.wikihow.com/Make-Liniment. Accessed 21 Apr. 2023.

Index

Made in the USA
Las Vegas, NV
21 November 2023

81292121R00125